Introduction to
Jewish and Catholic Bioethics

Moral Traditions Series
James F. Keenan, S.J., Editor

Introduction to
Jewish and Catholic Bioethics

A Comparative Analysis

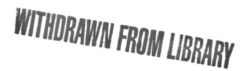

AARON L. MACKLER

Georgetown University Press
Washington, D.C.

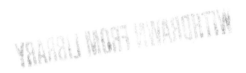
Georgetown University Press, Washington, D.C.
© 2003 by Georgetown University Press. All rights reserved.
Printed in the United States of America

10 9 8 7 6 5 4 3 2 1   2003

Library of Congress Cataloging-in-Publication Data

Mackler, Aaron L.
    Introduction to Jewish and Catholic Bioethics : a comparative analysis /
Aaron L. Mackler.
        p. cm. — (Moral traditions series)
Includes bibliographical references and index.
    ISBN 0-87840-146-6
    1. Medical ethics—Religious aspects—Judaism.   2. Medical ethics—
Religious aspects—Catholic Church.   3. Bioethics—Religious aspects—
Judaism.   4. Bioethics—Religious aspects—Catholic Church.   5. Religion and
ethics.   I. Title. II. Series.
    R725.55.M33 2003
    291.5'642—dc21

                                                         2003006938

Contents

Acknowledgments

THE DEVELOPMENT OF THIS BOOK HAS BEEN A LENGTHY and rewarding process, during which I have enjoyed the assistance of many people. My thinking about many of the issues discussed in this book was enriched by my work a decade ago as staff ethicist for the New York State Task Force on Life and the Law. The core argument of this work was presented in a paper delivered at the College Theology Society Annual Convention in 1996. This later was published as "Jewish and Roman Catholic Approaches to Bioethics: Convergence and Divergence in Method and Substance" in *Louvain Studies* 25 (2000): 3–22. An earlier version of chapter 7 originally was published as "Jewish and Roman Catholic Approaches to Access to Health Care and Rationing" in *Kennedy Institute of Ethics Journal* 11 (2001): 317–36. Significant material from chapter 2 is adapted from my introduction to *Life and Death Responsibilities in Jewish Biomedical Ethics* (New York: Jewish Theological Seminary of America, Finkelstein Institute, 2000), 1–14.

I am grateful for the support in developing this work provided by a summer stipend in 2000 from the National Endowment for the Humanities (no. FT-45174-00). I am thankful as well to Duquesne University for granting me a Presidential Scholarship stipend and for giving me a sabbatical leave that enabled me to devote extensive time to this project.

I have learned much from my colleagues and students at Duquesne University. I am particularly grateful to my colleagues in the Theology Department and in the graduate Health Care Ethics Program. Special thanks go to David F. Kelly, director of the Health Care Ethics Program, who has enriched my understanding of Roman Catholic bioethics and clinical health care ethics generally. He has offered crucial support from his original suggestion of the topic to reading the entire manuscript and offering valuable suggestions. Jim Hanigan, chair of the Theology Department, has encouraged my work and read the concluding chapter. My thinking on the issues of this book has been clarified and reshaped as well by my interaction with my students at Duquesne.

I also would like to express appreciation to my colleagues on the bioethics subcommittee of the Rabbinical Assembly's Committee on Jewish Law and Standards. In particular, Elliot Dorff has taught me much about Jewish bioethics and its methodology and provided important support at an early stage of the development of this project.

It has been a pleasure working with the staff at Georgetown University Press. Richard Brown, director, and Jim Keenan, editor of the Moral Traditions series, have offered astute comments on the manuscript and valuable advice on many aspects of the publication process.

During the period when I was revising the manuscript for this book I was hit by a car. I am grateful to the health care professionals who cared for me and afforded me a new perspective on health care and health care ethics. I am very thankful for the assistance given to my family and me by colleagues, friends, and family—especially my mother and my sister Rebecca.

I am pleased to have this opportunity to acknowledge my parents, Dr. Hyman and Ruth Mackler. Throughout my life they have been valued teachers and treasured sources of love and support. I also would like to express my appreciation to my children: Hannah, Joel, Daniel, and Ethan. I am grateful for their patience during my work on this project and for the happiness they add to my life.

Finally, I would like to express my debt of gratitude to my wife, Lorraine. She has offered helpful suggestions and personal support during the writing of this book. I am grateful for the countless ways in which she brings richness, joy, and love to my life. This book is dedicated in her honor.

Introduction

ONE OF THE CLASSIC, IF APOCRYPHAL, NARRATIVES ABOUT comparisons of religious traditions is related by Protestant ethicist James Gustafson. Three speakers were asked to offer Catholic, Jewish, and Protestant perspectives on a particular moral issue. The priest began, "The Church teaches that. . . ." The rabbi began, "The tradition teaches that. . . ." And the minister began, "Well, now I think that. . . ."[1]

A second anecdote arises from my work with an interdisciplinary and interreligious commission that addresses issues of bioethics and public policy. A Catholic attorney reported half-jokingly that he had asked his bishop what he might do if an issue arose for which he was uncertain about Catholic teaching. "If you want to know the Catholic position," he was told, "follow the rabbi"—referring to a very traditionalist Jewish member of the commission.

I use these anecdotes to illustrate three points. First, even an oversimplified account can be instructive. A full analysis of Jewish and Roman Catholic approaches to bioethics would require many books. The comparison in this book necessarily involves some broad strokes and simplifications. Nonetheless, I believe it conveys general characteristics that generally are accurate and important.

Second, as religious intellectual traditions with extensive histories of engagement with bioethics, Roman Catholicism and Judaism share important foundational elements and substantive positions. Nevertheless, as the first anecdote suggests, there are differences as well, including divergent methodologies. Jewish approaches generally are based on tradition, especially halakhah—a term meaning "path" or "way" and denoting Jewish law. Although Catholic moral approaches accord significant weight to tradition, more commonly they are centered on natural law, together with magisterial teaching.

1

Third, as the second anecdote suggests, there are significant and sometimes surprising points of convergence as well. In this book I explore similarities and differences between the two traditions, examining first general values and methodological concerns and then several substantive issues.

Overview

I begin with an overview of central values of the two traditions. At the most general level, the commonality of values is almost complete. Differences emerge within each tradition and in general tendencies between the traditions with regard to detailed specification and balancing of these fundamental values. In this introduction I focus on the common ground, leaving areas of divergence primarily for subsequent chapters.

In chapters 1 and 2 I sketch introductory overviews of methodological issues in Roman Catholic and Jewish ethics, respectively: the ways in which thinkers in each tradition build from general values to more particular and concrete guidance in addressing challenges within bioethics and other areas. Key issues that lead to divergences within each tradition, and to some extent between the traditions as a whole, include the construal of and weight given to reason and experience; understandings of tradition; and recognition of authority.

I then consider Jewish and Catholic views concerning five issues of bioethics: active euthanasia, forgoing life-sustaining treatment, abortion, in vitro fertilization, and justice and the allocation of health care resources. I attend to a broad range of thinkers and views, reflecting the diversity of influential writers in Catholic or Jewish discourse. Despite methodological differences at the theoretical level, theologians in both traditions frame issues in similar ways and identify similar sets of specific concerns. A spectrum of responses on these issues emerges in each tradition. The spectra overlap to a large extent on substantive issues as well as methodology. In some areas, such as those involving end-of-life decisions, the range of Jewish positions tends to overlap with and extend somewhat to the right of Catholic views—expressing greater reluctance to forgo life-sustaining treatment; on other issues, such as in vitro fertilization and other reproductive technologies, the Catholic range overlaps and extends somewhat to the right of Jewish views—expressing greater reluctance to allow these procedures. I explore some possible explanations for the remarkable convergence of the traditions and consider factors that may contribute to differences.

In the conclusion I look at general tendencies in the two traditions. I also briefly address the significance of convergence and divergence between these traditions for practical ethics, as practiced by moral thinkers within each faith community, and generally in the context of Western democracies such as the United States.[2]

Shared Values and Texts

Human Dignity and the Image of God

Significant points of convergence may be found at the level of general values. Both Judaism and Catholicism value the Hebrew Bible, or "Old Testament." Both find basic understandings of God and humanity reflected in this work, beginning with the creation narrative, that continue to be central to ethics today.[3] The book of Genesis teaches that God created humans in God's image.[4] Whether taken as a literal or mythic statement, this concept powerfully expresses the intrinsic value and dignity of each human being. The ancient Jewish sage, Ben Azzai, identified this proclamation as the greatest principle of the Torah (the Scripture and sacred "teaching" of Judaism).[5] Traditional and contemporary sources appropriately emphasize the importance of respect for persons (*kevod habriyot*). As expressed in a recent medical advance directive from the centrist Conservative movement of Judaism: "Life is a blessing and a gift from God. Each human being is valued as created *betzelem Elohim*, in God's image. Whatever the level of our physical and mental abilities, whatever the extent of our dependence on others, each person has intrinsic dignity and value in God's eyes."[6]

Similar understandings are articulated by Catholic moral theologians, including the late Richard McCormick. "God is the author and preserver of life. We are 'made in His image.' Thus life is a gift, a trust. It has great worth because of the value He is placing in it."[7] In this statement McCormick follows the Second Vatican Council's *Gaudium et Spes*, which begins its discussion of "the dignity of the human person" by considering "man as the image of God":

For sacred Scripture teaches that man was created "to the image of God," as able to know and love his creator, and as set by him over all earthly creatures that he might rule over them, and make use of them, while glorifying God. "What is man that thou are mindful of him, and the son of man that thou dost care for him? Yet thou hast made him little less than God, and dost crown him with glory and honor."[8]

Body and Soul

For theologians in each tradition, God's creation and ongoing concern endows with value the full human person, a unity of body and soul. Historically, some thinkers in each tradition have disparaged the body as an encumbrance or even prison for the spirit or soul. Most contemporary thinkers would agree that the human person is more than physical, and many would accord a certain priority to the soul or spiritual aspect of the person.[9] Regardless, theologians of both traditions overwhelmingly would endorse the understanding of *Gaudium et Spes*:

> Man, though made of body and soul, is a unity. Through his very bodily condition he sums up in himself the elements of the material world. . . . For this reason man may not despise his bodily life. Rather he is obliged to regard his body as good and to hold it in honor since God has created it.[10]

Elliot Dorff posits as "fundamental beliefs underlying Jewish medical ethics" both that "the human being is an integrated whole" and that "the body is morally neutral and potentially good." The body is subject to misuse but also "can and should be used for divine purposes. . . . Within [appropriate] constraints, the body's pleasures are God-given and not to be shunned, for to do so would be an act of ingratitude toward our Creator."[11]

Life

The value of life is powerful—and generally decisive—in the Jewish tradition. Saving a life (*pikuah nefesh*) justifies virtually any action that otherwise would be prohibited by the tradition, such as eating on the fast day of Yom Kippur. According to Jewish law, there are only three exceptions to the overriding value of saving life: murder, idolatry, and the illicit sexual relations of adultery or incest. Otherwise, the value of saving life is always decisive.[12] Furthermore, violating provisions of Jewish law to save a life is not only permitted but required; Judaism teaches the obligation to help others in need and, especially, to save life. A classical statement is found in the book of Leviticus (19:16): "You shall not stand idly by the blood of your neighbor." A Talmudic passage supports this mandate by an appeal to the creation narrative of Genesis. Why does the Bible present God as beginning the creation of humanity with a single person? "To teach you that anyone who destroys a single person from the children of man [Adam] is considered by Scripture as if he destroyed an entire world, and whoever sustains a single person from the children of man is considered as if he sustained an entire world."[13] In the words of the medieval physician and rabbi Moses Naḥmanides: "Saving life is a great mitzvah [commandment]. Who approaches it with alacrity is praised, who hesitates is despicable, who questions it is guilty of murder, and certainly so, one who despairs and does not do it."[14] The crucial importance of saving life is affirmed by theologians in all branches of contemporary Judaism.[15]

Catholic thinkers assert esteem for the value of life as well. In the 1995 *Evangelium Vitae*, Pope John Paul II affirms that "life is always a good." "To defend and promote life, to show reverence and love for it, is a task which God entrusts to every man." Accordingly, "we are all committed to ensure to our neighbor, that his or her life may be always defended and promoted, especially when it is weak or threatened. It is not only a personal but a social concern which we must all foster: a concern to make unconditional respect for human life the foundation of a renewed society." "In giving life to man, God demands that he love, respect, and promote life. The gift becomes a commandment."[16] Catholic theologians overwhelmingly agree that life is a great, basic, and sacred value. Catholic thinkers also note that physical life is not an absolute good: For example, martyrdom would justify the sacrifice of one's life.[17] Jewish authorities would agree that in some sense life is not the highest good and that in extreme cases it would be appropriate to accept death for the sake of martyrdom, or sanctification of the divine name (*kiddush Hashem*).[18] Within the broad agreement of the two traditions, there are some differences in nuance and emphasis, as I discuss in subsequent chapters.[19]

Imitation of God

A central call in each tradition is to follow in God's paths and, indeed, to imitate God; in Christianity this call typically is expressed as imitation of Christ, or "the imitation of God in Christ."[20] The Letter to the Ephesians (5:1–2) proclaims, "So be imitators of God, as beloved children, and live in love, as Christ loved us." Richard McCormick writes that "the moral life reproduces in the Christian the moral attitudes of Christ himself. This will be a following of Christ, which means to love God by keeping his commandments, and to love one's neighbor as Jesus loved us, even to death." Likewise the "Ethical and Religious Directives for Catholic Health Care Services" of the National Conference of Catholic Bishops speaks of service to the sick "in faithful imitation of Jesus Christ."[21]

Jewish views of the imitation of God go back to Leviticus (19:1): "The Lord said to Moses, 'Speak to the whole Israelite community, and tell them: Be holy, for I, the Lord your God, am holy.'" Traditional sources understand the imitation of God as a mitzvah and as the ground for particular moral obligations.[22] The call to imitate God is understood primarily in terms of imitating God's actions and attributes, though for some thinkers it also entails becoming like God. "Loving-kindness above all is the goal of all human action, and by practicing it man becomes like his Creator and fulfills the *imitatio Dei*."[23]

The Talmud expresses both the paradox of attempting to imitate the transcendent God and the significance of deeds of kindness and mercy. The Talmud asks: What could it mean when the Bible commands, "walk after the Lord your God"? Is it possible for a human to follow after the Divine Presence? As the Bible proclaims, "The Lord your God is a consuming fire":

> Rather, we are called to follow after the attributes of the Holy One, Blessed be He. Just as He clothes the naked, as it is written, "The Lord God made garments of skin for Adam and his wife and clothed them," so you should clothe the naked. The Holy One visited the ill, as it is written, "The Lord appeared to [Abraham] by the oaks of Mamre" [as he was recuperating from circumcision]; so also you should visit the ill. The Holy One comforted mourners, as it is written, "After the death of Abraham, God blessed his son Isaac," so you should comfort mourners. The Holy One buried the dead, as it

is written, "He buried [Moses] in the valley," so also you should bury the dead.[24]

Love of Neighbor

Both Roman Catholicism and Judaism accord special esteem to the commandment, "Love your neighbor as yourself." This commandment, appearing first in Leviticus, is identified by Jesus as one of the two greatest commandments (along with the call of Deuteronomy to love God). Similarly, Rabbi Akiba viewed this commandment as the greatest principle of the Torah.[25] Catholic thinkers Benedict Ashley and Kevin O'Rourke write that "the essence of Christian life is the sharing by grace in this love of God, by which we love him and one another." Similarly, McCormick observes that love, or charity, is "the principle of the moral life" and the "form of the virtues."[26] Jewish writers understand the commandment to call for deeds of care and compassion and for cultivation of appropriate spiritual attitudes.[27] Jewish and Catholic writers state that love and compassion are (or should be) distinguishing characteristics of members of their faith community.[28]

Divine Sovereignty and Human Stewardship

Each tradition includes both calls to human activity and cautions to avoid usurping God's sovereignty. The book of Genesis (1–3) proclaims God's sovereignty over the universe and his setting of restrictions on the legitimate scope of human activity. At the same time, God charges humanity to work and to subdue and to have dominion over the world (Gen. 1:28, 2:15). David Kelly identifies two complementary theological themes in the Roman Catholic tradition. One "concerns God's dominion over human life, and purports to judge concerning the obligation of men and women . . . to respect God's sovereignty." This theme is complemented by the responsibility of human activity. The two themes are

> two aspects of one central theological axis: What is one's relationship to the creator? To what extent is one a creature; to what extent a co-creator, or at least a co-agent with God? . . . Is it God's will that we try to "create a better world," that we join with our creator as

co-sovereigns over life, that we eliminate suffering (and even death) to the extent that we can? Or is it rather God's will that we respect the sovereignty of God alone, that we accept our position in resignation to God's will?[29]

In each tradition, although respect for God's sovereignty is powerful there is some tendency for the active side of the balance to predominate. As the New Testament's Letter of James (2:15–17) proclaims, "If a brother or sister has nothing to wear and has no food for the day, and one of you says to them, 'Go in peace, keep warm, and eat well,' but you do not give them the necessities of the body, what good is it? So also faith of itself, if it does not have works, is dead." Pope John Paul II writes that the human, "created in the image of God, shares by his work in the activity of the creator and that, within the limits of his own human capabilities, man in a sense continues to develop that activity, and perfects it."[30] Similarly, Judaism asserts human responsibility for reverent but active partnership with God in completing the works of creation and improving the world (*tikkun ha'olam*).[31]

In sum, both traditions value the world as created by God—and thus basically good—yet understand the world as we know it to be less than perfect. Accordingly, in the words of the bishops' "Ethical and Religious Directives," humans are to exercise

> stewardship over all material creation that should neither abuse nor squander nature's resources. Through science the human race comes to understand God's wonderful work; and through technology it must conserve, protect and perfect nature in harmony with God's purposes. Health care professionals pursue a special vocation to share in carrying forth God's life-giving and healing work.[32]

Healing

Over the course of history, each tradition has experienced debate about the implications for human healing of the commitments to respect divine sovereignty and to exercise active stewardship. Indeed, the Bible depicts God as purposefully causing illness (as well as famine and other forms of human suffering) and providing healing.[33] As framed by David Kelly, the question arises, "what is the relationship between divine and human causality? . . . Is the healing of disease a cooperation with God's creative plan, or is it rather a contradiction of that plan, a usurpation of God's sovereignty, a removing of what God has sent?"[34] A minority of thinkers in each tradition historically expressed doubt about the legitimacy of much health care. In the Middle Ages, Jewish thinker Abraham Ibn Ezra endorsed only the healing of external injuries. Moses Nahmanides regarded the practice of medicine as a concession to human weakness because the faithful ideally would rely on God alone.[35] Some Catholic authorities, including Tertullian and St. Bernard of Clairvaux, rejected medical care.[36]

Nevertheless, throughout their history—and overwhelmingly in the past century—the two traditions have accepted and valued health care as a responsible exercise of human stewardship. Such activity is compatible with and, in fact, demanded by respect for divine sovereignty. "Because God owns our bodies, we are required to help other people escape sickness, injury, and death. . . . We are all under the divine imperative to help God preserve and protect what is God's."[37] Although various explanations have been suggested for the mysteries of theodicy and divine providence, the overwhelming consensus of the traditions is that God has entrusted humans with the power and responsibility to feed the hungry, comfort the afflicted, and heal the sick. As the classical Jewish code, the *Shulḥan Arukh*, frames it, God has both given permission to heal and imposed the obligation to do so. In the Jewish tradition, the authority and responsibility to heal has been understood to be grounded in biblical mandates to heal the injured (Exodus 21:19); to restore that which has been lost—construed to include lost health and function (Deuteronomy 22:2); and to love one's neighbor as oneself (Leviticus 19:18).[38]

Similarly, Catholic authorities affirm that healing is an appropriate and mandated human activity that expresses love of neighbor.[39] Kelly summarizes Thomas Aquinas's understanding of divine sovereignty and causality: "Though God is the ultimate, or primary cause, God works through created secondary causes which we can study and learn to manipulate. These are patterns embedded by God in creation, patterns which God expects us to learn about and to work with."[40] Similarly, Noam Zohar presents the position of Moses Maimonides:

"God acts in the world chiefly or even solely through natural causality. Sound medicine, like sound technology in general, is itself an instance of God's providence."[41]

Community

Although each individual has intrinsic value, humans are essentially social as well. Thomas Aquinas asserts that "living in society" represents a basic human good, toward which humans have a natural inclination; "whatever this [inclination] involves is a matter of natural law, for instance, that a man should . . . not offend others with whom he ought to live in civility." Among contemporary thinkers, Louis Janssens affirms as a fundamental dimension of the human person that "human beings are essentially directed toward each other." Drawing on *Gaudium et Spes*, he continues: "Human persons are not only essentially social beings because they are open to each other in the I-Thou relationship, but also because they need to live in social groups and thus in appropriate structures and institutions. We must live in society."[42] As Richard McCormick adds, "our well-being is interdependent. It cannot be conceived of or realistically pursued independently of the good of others."[43] Jewish thinkers of diverse viewpoints agree that one's identity is in part formed by the community of which one is a member. As Reform (left wing) thinker Eugene Borowitz observes, the Jewish tradition teaches that human nature is social; even with the insights of modernity, it remains true that an individual's identity is and should be shaped largely by the community of which one is part.[44]

A traditional text uses a story to illustrate the interdependence of individuals. Some people were sitting in a boat, and one of them took a drill and began to bore a hole under his seat. His companions protested, "Why are you doing that?" The man replied, "What does this have to do with you? Am I not drilling under my own seat?" They replied, "You are going to let the water in and sink the boat!"[45]

The social nature of humans is highlighted for both Judaism and Roman Catholicism, whose members see themselves as part of a covenanted community: the Jew who is a member of the community of Israel, the Catholic who is a member of the Church and through that part of the people of God and body of Christ. As Richard McCormick writes, "In the Judeo-Christian story, God relates to and makes covenants with a people. . . . As Christians, we live, move, and have our Christian being as a believing group, an *ecclesia*. Our being in Christ is a shared being."[46] Similarly, Judaism teaches that Jews, as part of the community of Israel, participate in a communal covenantal relationship with God.[47]

Historically both Judaism and Roman Catholicism have appreciated the richness of life in the community of faith, while recognizing the intrinsic value of, and ethical responsibilities toward, all human persons—including those outside the believing community. Each community has faced distinctive challenges in modernity in formulating and living out an ethic that is both concerned with and respectful toward people outside the community.

Jewish ethics historically focused on the responsibilities of Jews to fellow Jews. This focus reflected not only a theoretical valuing of the community but also the practical social conditions under which Jews lived. For most of Judaism's history, Jews lived in independent Jewish communities or semiautonomous communities within a broader corporate state. For most of the past 2,000 years, Jews were discriminated against to one extent or another, oppressed or at best tolerated by what was experienced as an external, non-Jewish world. The tradition includes some discussions of the ethical responsibilities of all persons, understood through a model of God's covenant with "the children of Noah" (i.e., with all of humanity).[48] Most theologians have endorsed the Talmud's statement that not only Jews but righteous individuals of all nations will enjoy the salvation of a portion in the world to come. Historically, ethical responsibilities of Jews toward non-Jews were recognized; these responsibilities tended to fit a model of a responsible but distant ethics of strangers—reflecting the real-life context of the time. Traditional sources instructed that non-Jews together with Jews should receive financial support for the poor, visiting of the ill, and other works of philanthropy.[49] The extent to which these mandates were carried out, like relations between Jews and non-Jews generally, varied greatly.

Since about 1800, large and growing numbers of Jews have had the status of individual citizens within secular states. The advent of modernity entailed radically new ideas and a radically new life situation. Modern thinkers increasingly came to see in the Bible's account of "having God begin humankind with but one pair of people an early intuition of the truth that all ethics is necessarily universal. Put symbolically, one Divine Parent meant that all human beings have familial obligations to one another."[50] Most contemporary thinkers assert special responsibilities for members of one's community (the Jewish community, as well as local and national communities), in addition to important responsibilities for all of humanity.

From its early years, Christianity has expressed concern with all humans. Throughout the Middle Ages and beyond, this breadth of concern was reinforced by the position of Roman Catholic Christianity as the dominant and established religion of nations. At times, however, this extensive concern was accompanied by intolerance for persons who did not share Catholic Christian faith—religious minorities living within predominantly Catholic states or those in foreign countries.[51] Official church documents and individual theologians agreed that "there is no salvation outside the Church," that other religions are false, and that error has no rights to respect.[52] The Second Vatican Council represented a landmark in a dramatic process of growing acceptance of the value of religious liberty and respect for other faiths. The same Council articulated a powerful engagement with the challenges of the contemporary world and "solidarity of the church with the whole human family."[53]

Justice

Both Judaism and Roman Catholicism teach the crucial importance of justice. This commitment flows from both appreciation of the importance of the community and recognition of the intrinsic value of each individual. Both traditions understand God as manifesting special concern for weak and vulnerable persons and mandating that humans also act with such concern for the weak and vulnerable among us. Judaism developed the Hebrew Bible's value of justice and its institutions for the support of the poor into a system of *tzedakah*—literally meaning justice and signifying aid for the poor. Similarly, Roman Catholicism teaches the value of justice and the importance of charitable support for persons in need. Both traditions mandate (as necessary but not sufficient) what the National Conference of Catholic Bishops terms "basic justice"—"the establishment of a floor of material well-being on which all can stand." Society must go beyond this basic justice to include "social justice, [which] implies that persons have an obligation to be active and productive participants in the life of society and that society has a duty to enable them to participate in this way."[54] I explore understandings of justice and its implications for health care in chapter 7.

Family

Both Roman Catholicism and Judaism value the family. Marriage is supported by values of both loving companionship and procreation. Both values may be found in the creation narrative of Genesis. God blesses the first humans, "Be fruitful and multiply." After creating Adam, God observed that "it is not good for man to be alone" and created Eve, his true companion. "Hence a man leaves his father and mother and clings to his wife, so that they become one flesh." Both traditions value children as a blessing for their parents and for the broader community.[55]

McCormick suggests as themes of Catholic ethics the bond between "life giving and love making," in sexuality and in marriage generally, and "heterosexual, permanent marriage as normative."[56] Traditionally, these themes have represented the ideal for both religions. Diverse views may be found within each tradition regarding situations that vary from the ideal—for example, if a couple is infertile and requires the use of artificial reproductive technologies to have a child. I discuss this issue in greater detail in chapter 6.[57]

Autonomy

Both Roman Catholicism and Judaism value autonomy and respect for the conscientious choices of individuals. As the Second Vatican Council proclaimed, "the human person has a right to religious freedom. Freedom of this kind means that all men should be immune from coercion on the part of individuals, social groups and every human power so that, within due limits, nobody is forced to act against his convictions."[58] Within Judaism, the value of autonomy is emphasized most strongly by Reform thinkers, though it is recognized by others as well.[59] In the health care setting, the value of autonomy supports respect for the choices of individual patients, empowering patients to offer or withhold their informed consent for treatment. As expressed by Orthodox (right wing) rabbi Irving Greenberg, "the patient himself must have a role in therapy. The patient is in the image of God; thus the greater the role in the patient's own therapy, the greater the patient's own dignity."[60] Likewise, Ashley and O'Rourke affirm a "principle of free and informed consent."[61]

Religious thinkers differ among themselves—and as a group tend to differ from secular writers—on the specification and balancing of the value of autonomy. Writers note that all of the ethical values of the tradition—not only autonomy—must be respected, so there are limits to the appropriate range of patient choices. For example, Orthodox rabbi J. David Bleich recognizes liberty as an important ethical value but argues that in case of conflict it should give way to the cardinal principle of the preservation of life.[62] Ashley and O'Rourke recognize a "principle of well-formed conscience" while noting a responsibility "to use our freedom in accordance with objective truth"—including what they (following official Catholic teaching) present as the objective requirements of morality.[63] I consider Jewish and Roman Catholic understandings of the appropriate extent of individual authority in chapters 1 and 2, as well as throughout the book.

Summary

In this introduction I have noted extensive agreement between Roman Catholicism and Judaism with regard to fundamental ethical values and the worldviews that shape and support those values. Of course, there are major differences between the traditions as well—in the way the shared values are understood as well as on other points. Although I have purposefully glossed over these differences in this initial presentation, they are apparent throughout this book. Yet this survey of common ground shared by the traditions places those differences in perspective. Some of the central foundational values are articulated by Conservative rabbi Seymour Siegel, in a statement presented by James McCartney as a summary of Catholic views as well:

> In conclusion, we are guided by the principle that life is precious; that we are bidden to preserve and guard our health; that we are bidden to intervene in nature to raise the human estate; and that our lives

are not our own, but are part of the legacy bequeathed to us by the Creator. In our community there are differences of approach and interpretation. Let us discuss these issues with reason and prayerful dialogue, hoping that God will guide us in our decision-making so that we can better serve Him and our fellowman.[64]

This book reflects that spirit.

Notes

1. James M. Gustafson, *Protestant and Roman Catholic Ethics: Prospects for Rapprochement* (Chicago: University of Chicago Press, 1978), 4–5.

2. In this book I consider writers from the United States most extensively, although I also give attention to thinkers in Europe and Israel. Accordingly, the conclusions of this work are established most clearly for Western nations, especially the United States—although I believe that they remain valuable for general comparison of Judaism and Roman Catholicism.

3. Louis E. Newman, *Past Imperatives: Studies in the History and Theory of Jewish Ethics* (Albany: State University of New York Press, 1999), 108; Richard A. McCormick, *Health and Medicine in the Catholic Tradition* (New York: Crossroad, 1987), 48–50; John Paul II, *Laborem Exercens: On Human Work [LE]* (Washington, D.C.: United States Catholic Conference, 1981), n. 4, p. 9.

4. Gen. 1:27; similarly Gen. 5:1, 9:6.

5. Genesis Rabbah 24:7, *Sifra* 89b, in C. G. Montefiore and H. Loewe, *A Rabbinic Anthology* (New York: Schocken, 1974), 172. As Rabbi Tanhuma notes, to insult another person thus is to insult a being created in God's image (Genesis Rabbah 24:7). On the Torah, see chapter 2.

6. Aaron L. Mackler, ed., "Jewish Medical Directives for Health Care," in *Life and Death Responsibilities in Jewish Biomedical Ethics*, ed. Aaron L. Mackler (New York: Jewish Theological Seminary Press, Finkelstein Institute, 2000), 367. See also Elliot N. Dorff, *Matters of Life and Death: A Jewish Approach to Modern Medical Ethics* (Philadelphia: Jewish Publication Society, 1998), 18–20.

7. Richard A. McCormick, "How to Draw Guidance from a Heritage: A Catholic Approach to Mortal Choices," in *A Time to Be Born and a Time to Die: The Ethics of Choice*, ed. Barry S. Kogan (New York: Aldine de Gruyter, 1991), 234.

8. *Gaudium et Spes: Pastoral Constitution on the Church in the Modern World [GS]*, 12, in *Vatican Council II: The Conciliar and Post Conciliar*

Documents, new rev. ed., ed. Austin Flannery (Northport, N.Y.: Costello, 1996), p. 913, quoting Psalm 8. "Being in the image of God the human individual possesses the dignity of a person, who is not just something, but someone"; *Catechism of the Catholic Church* (Mission Hills, Calif.: Benziger, 1994), n. 357, p. 91.

9. Among many possible examples, John Mahoney observes that "for Augustine, with his Neoplatonist background, man is viewed as 'a rational soul using a mortal earthly body'"; *The Making of Moral Theology: A Study of the Roman Catholic Tradition* (New York: Clarendon Press, Oxford University Press, 1987), 55, quoting *De moribus ecclesiae catholicae* 1, 27. See also Dorff, *Matters of Life and Death*, 20–26; Harold M. Schulweis, "Judaism: From Either/Or to Both/And," in *Contemporary Jewish Ethics and Morality: A Reader*, ed. Elliot N. Dorff and Louis E. Newman (New York: Oxford University Press, 1995), 25–37.

10. *GS* 14, in *Vatican Council II*, 914–15. See also Benedict M. Ashley and Kevin D. O'Rourke, *Health Care Ethics: A Theological Analysis*, 4th ed. (Washington, D.C.: Georgetown University Press, 1997), 166, 173; Louis Janssens, "Artificial Insemination: Ethical Considerations," *Louvain Studies* 7 (1980): 5–6, who observes that "the person is a subject in corporeality . . . corporeal and spiritual, nonetheless a singular being." In discussing the goodness of the body, *Gaudium et Spes* proclaims that God "will raise it up on the last day." Physical resurrection is a traditional Jewish belief—maintained by some Jews in a literal sense and understood by others in a mythical sense as a symbolic affirmation of the value of bodily life; others simply reject it. See Neil Gillman, *The Death of Death: Resurrection and Immortality in Jewish Thought* (Woodstock, Vt.: Jewish Lights, 1997), 215–74; Will Herberg, *Judaism and Modern Man: An Interpretation of Jewish Religion* (New York: Farrar Straus and Young, 1951; Atheneum, 1970), 211–39. After affirming the goodness of the body, *Gaudium et Spes* continues to state that because of sin, man "finds by experience that his body is in revolt." Although sin is an important concern in Jewish theology, the image of the body in revolt would be uncommon among contemporary Jewish thinkers.

11. Dorff, *Matters of Life and Death*, 20–26. See also Newman, *Past Imperatives* (110), who observes that "as understood by Jewish authorities, the sacredness of human life inheres in the human being as a whole, both body and soul." Dorff, *Matters of Life and Death* (24), presents this positive approach to the body as contrasting sharply with Christian—in particular Roman Catholic—beliefs, which depict "the body as a negative part of us to be suppressed as much as possible. Thus in Catholic and many Protestant sources, the ideal Christian is the ascetic, who eschews the pleasures of sex,

food, and possessions as much as possible." I agree with Dorff that Catholic esteem for "the more perfect way" of the monastic or religious life, with vows of poverty and celibacy, does contrast with Judaism. Nevertheless, especially in contemporary thought, the basis for this is more complex than simple denial of the body. Both body-affirming and more ascetic strands may be found in each tradition. See Schulweis, "Judaism," 27–29; James P. Hanigan, *As I Have Loved You: The Challenge of Christian Ethics* (Mahwah, N.J.: Paulist, 1986), 190–208.

12. See Talmud, *Yoma* 82a–85b, *Sanhedrin* 74a. The sins of murder, idolatry, and adultery are regarded as especially grievous within Christian tradition, as noted by Mahoney, *The Making of Moral Theology*, 3–4; John Paul II, *Evangelium Vitae: The Gospel of Life [EV]* (Washington, D.C.: United States Catholic Conference, 1995), n. 54, p. 97.

13. Talmud, *Sanhedrin* 37a (Mishnah *Sanhedrin* 4:5). This passage may be familiar to readers because of its use in the movie *Schindler's List*.

14. Naḥmanides, *Torat Ha'adam*, quoted by Avram Israel Reisner, "Care for the Terminally Ill: Halakhic Concepts and Values," in *Life and Death Responsibilities*, 239.

15. Newman, *Past Imperatives* (108–9), begins his summary of major principles of Jewish ethics by stating, "That human life is sacred means, in the first place, that it possesses intrinsic and infinite value. Its value is absolute, not susceptible to quantification and not relative to the value of anything extrinsic to it. . . . The sanctity of life generates a second major principle of Jewish ethics, that the preservation of life is the highest moral imperative." See also J. David Bleich, "The Obligation to Heal in the Jewish Tradition," in *Jewish Bioethics*, ed. Fred Rosner and J. David Bleich (New York: Sanhedrin, 1979), 17; Dorff, *Matters of Life and Death*, 15–20; Eugene B. Borowitz, *Exploring Jewish Ethics* (Detroit: Wayne State University Press, 1990), 20–21.

16. *EV*, nn. 34, 42, 77, 52; pp. 60, 73, 140, 93.

17. *EV*, n. 47, p. 83; Congregation for the Doctrine of the Faith, "Declaration on Euthanasia," *Origins* 10 (1980): 155; McCormick, *Health and Medicine*, 51–52.

18. See Baruch A. Brody, "A Historical Introduction to Jewish Casuistry on Suicide and Euthanasia," in *Suicide and Euthanasia: Historical and Contemporary Themes*, ed. Baruch A. Brody (Dordrecht, Netherlands: Kluwer, 1989), 39–75.

19. See especially chapter 4 and the conclusion. There are differences in degree in the value accorded to life in this world relative to life eternal or in the world to come. Some people have claimed that Judaism is a "this-worldly"

religion and Christianity "other-worldly." Although this claim is oversimplified, it does contain an element of truth. For many Catholic theologians, the central narrative of Jesus's death and resurrection has relativized the life of this world. Life in this world clearly is subordinated to spiritual development and life eternal. See *EV*, n. 47, p. 83; McCormick, *Health and Medicine*, 51–52; Ashley and O'Rourke, *Health Care Ethics*, 396–97; *Catechism of the Catholic Church*, nn. 1005–20, pp. 262–66; Bernard Häring, *The Law of Christ*, vol. 1, trans. Edwin G. Kaiser (Westminster, Md.: Newman, 1963), 141–43.

Although Jewish views on this subject are complex and varied, few Jewish theologians would put things quite the same way. A typical Jewish understanding is that this world and life eternal represent two goods that are each basic and incommensurable, neither serving only instrumentally for the other. As expressed by Rabbi Jacob in the third-century Mishnah (*Avot* 4:21), "Better is one hour of repentance and good deeds in this world than all of life eternal in the world to come; and better is one hour of bliss in the world to come than all of life in this world." See Schulweis, "Judaism," 25–29; Dorff, *Matters of Life and Death*, 30–31.

20. The phrase is used by Bernard Häring in characterizing the view of Clement of Alexandria (*The Law of Christ*, 1: 7). For Häring (*The Law of Christ*, 1: 51), "The foundation for the imitation of Christ is the incorporation of the disciple in Christ through grace. Imitation of Christ in our lives is accomplished through activity of love and obedience in objective union with Christ. Imitation binds us to the word of Christ: in His grace, in the gift of love, Christ binds us to Himself. In love we unite ourselves with His Person, the Incarnate Word. Our obedience unites us with Him through the following of His example eloquently inviting us to imitate Him."

21. McCormick, *Health and Medicine*, 34; National Conference of Catholic Bishops, "Ethical and Religious Directives for Catholic Health Care Services," *Origins* 24 (1994): 452. *Gaudium et Spes* proclaims, "whoever follows Christ the perfect man becomes himself more a man" (n. 41, *Vatican Council II*, p. 941). See also National Conference of Catholic Bishops, "Pastoral Letter on Health and Health Care," *Origins* 11 (1981): 396–402.

22. David S. Shapiro, "The Doctrine of the Image of God and *Imitatio Dei*," in *Contemporary Jewish Ethics*, ed. Menachem Marc Kellner (New York: Sanhedrin, 1978), 135–36. In his code of Jewish law, the *Mishneh Torah*, Moses Maimonides writes, "The sages taught, 'even as God is called gracious, so be you gracious; even as He is called merciful, so be you merciful; even as He is called holy, so be you holy.' Thus too the prophets described the Almighty by all the various attributes, 'long-suffering and abounding in

kindness, righteous and upright, perfect, mighty and powerful,' and so forth, to teach that these qualities are good and right and that a human being should cultivate them, and thus imitate God, as far as he can" (The Laws of Ethics [*De'ot*] 1: 6; in *A Maimonides Reader*, ed. Isadore Twersky [New York: Behrman House, 1972], 53).

23. Shapiro, "The Doctrine of the Image of God and *Imitatio Dei*,"133. See also Martin Buber, "Imitatio Dei," in Dorff and Newman, *Contemporary Jewish Ethics*, 152–61.

24. *Sotah* 14a, quoting Deut. 13:5, 4:24; Gen. 3 21, 18:1, 25:11, Deut. 34:6.

25. Lev. 19:18, Deut. 6:4–5, Mt. 22:36–39, Mk. 12:28–31; *Sifra* 89b.

26. Ashley and O'Rourke, *Health Care Ethics*, 214; McCormick, *Health and Medicine*, 33–34. See similarly Hanigan, *As I Have Loved You,* 7–9, and numerous other works.

27. Louis Jacobs, *Jewish Values* (Hartford, Conn.: Hartmore House, 1960), 118–44.

28. McCormick, *Health and Medicine*, 34, citing John 13:35; Jacobs, *Jewish Values,* 135, citing Talmud, *Yevamot* 79a, *Betzah* 32b. Agreement on the importance of love of neighbor does not prevent some Jewish or Roman Catholic thinkers from arguing that the understanding and practice of neighbor love in their tradition is superior to that found in the other. As writers point out about their own and/or the other tradition, both traditions have been inconsistent historically with regard to the scope accorded to love of neighbor, in terms of both theoretical understanding and practice. Leviticus (19:34) includes a parallel injunction to love the stranger as oneself. Historically, love of neighbor often has been understood primarily in the context of relations with fellow members of the faith community, although—especially in recent decades—there has been some attention to responsibilities of love for all humans. See, e.g., Ernst Simon, "The Neighbor (Re'a) Whom We Shall Love," in *Modern Jewish Ethics: Theory and Practice*, ed. Marvin Fox (Columbus: Ohio State University Press, 1975), 29–56; Karl Rahner, *The Love of Jesus and the Love of Neighbor*, trans. Robert Barr (New York: Crossroad, 1983), who understands love of neighbor in terms of the fraternity of Christian communion.

29. David F. Kelly, *The Emergence of Roman Catholic Medical Ethics in North America* (New York: Edward Mellen Press, 1979), 233, 436. In support of the theme of resignation, Kelly adds the understanding that "our suffering love is redemptive if actively joined to the redemptive suffering of Jesus." He identifies an additional principle of "the redemptive meaning of suffering."

30. *LE*, n. 25, p. 53. Ashley and O'Rourke, *Health Care Ethics*, 202, articulate a "Principle of Stewardship and Creativity": "The gifts of multidimensional human nature and its natural environment should be used with profound respect for their intrinsic teleology."

31. See Talmud, *Shabbat* 10a, 119b. Irving Greenberg writes, "There is a covenant between God and humanity. . . . The human role in this covenant is to perfect the world which was brought into being by God . . . To perfect the world means that the human is called upon not to accept the world as it is, but to improve it and to complete it. . . . The key to constructive use of power is partnership" ("Toward a Covenantal Ethic of Medicine," in *Jewish Values in Bioethics*, ed. Levi Meier [New York: Human Sciences Press, 1986], 128–34.

32. National Conference of Catholic Bishops, "Directives," 452, citing Genesis 1:26.

33. See, e.g., Leviticus 26:14–16, Deuteronomy 28, Exodus 15:26, II Chronicles 16:12; and generally Dorff, 26–27, and David F. Kelly, *A Theological Basis for Health Care and Health Care Ethics* (Milwaukee, Wisc.: National Association of Catholic Chaplains, 1985), 41.

34. Kelly, *Theological Basis for Health Care*, 39–40.

35. Noam J. Zohar, *Alternatives in Jewish Bioethics* (Albany: State University of New York Press, 1997), 19–29; Dorff, *Matters of Life and Death*, 26; Immanuel Jakobovits, *Jewish Medical Ethics*, rev. ed. (New York: Bloch, 1975), 4–6. Both Naḥmanides and Ibn Ezra practiced as physicians, so their objections seem more theoretical than practical.

36. See Kelly, *Theological Basis for Health Care*, 42. As recently as 1829, Pope Leo XII rejected vaccination against smallpox. "Whoever allows himself to be vaccinated ceases to be a child of God. Smallpox is a judgment of God, the vaccination is a challenge toward heaven" (see Janssens, "Artificial Insemination," 11, citing A. Jeannière, "Corps maliéable," *Cahiers Laënnec* 29 [1968]: 94).

37. Dorff, *Matters of Life and Death*, 26. Similarly, because of God's ultimate sovereignty humans have an obligation to preserve their own health; see Dorff, *Matters of Life and Death*, 18; Maimonides, *Mishneh Torah*, "Laws of Ethics," 3–4; Ashley and O'Rourke, *Health Care Ethics*, 42–44. Edmund D. Pellegrino writes, "A Christian philosophy of healing must begin with God, the creator of human life, the giver of a precious gift, the creator of a human soul united with a body. Those who receive this gift inherit the duties of stewardship—duties to preserve the well-functioning of the soul, body, and mind, never to abuse them, to heal them when they are ill and healing is possible, and to care for and sustain them when cure is not possible" ("Healing and Being Healed: A Christian Perspective," in *Jewish and Catholic*

Bioethics: An Ecumenical Dialogue, ed. Edmund D. Pellegrino and Alan I. Faden [Washington, D.C.: Georgetown University Press, 1999], 117).

38. See Joseph Karo, *Shulḥan Arukh*, *Yoreh De'ah* 336:1; David M. Feldman, *Health and Medicine in the Jewish Tradition* (New York: Crossroad, 1986), 15–21; Bleich, "The Obligation to Heal," 20–28; Fred Rosner, "The Imperative to Heal in Traditional Judaism," in *Jewish and Catholic Bioethics*, 99–105. One classical narrative depicts two rabbis offering medical advice to an ill individual, only to have the patient accuse them of interfering with God's will in making the person ill. The rabbis asked the man, a farmer, why he interfered with the God-given state of his vineyard by fertilizing and weeding. When he responded that crops would not grow well without human care, the rabbis replied: "Just as plants, if not weeded, fertilized, and plowed, will not grow and bring forth fruits, so with the human body. The fertilizer is the medicine and the means of healing, and the tiller of the earth is the physician" (*Midrash Temurah*, translation based on Feldman, *Health and Medicine in the Jewish Tradition*, 16). Traditional sources reflect appreciation for the powerful and divinely mandated value of the physician's service. As expressed in a physician's prayer attributed to Moses Maimonides: "Inspire me with love for my art and for Your creatures. Do not allow thirst for profit, ambition for renown and admiration, to interfere with my profession, for these are the enemies of truth and of love for mankind and they can lead astray in the great task of attending to the welfare of Your creatures. Preserve the strength of my body and of my soul that they ever be ready to cheerfully help and support rich and poor, good and bad, enemy as well as friend. In the sufferer let me see only the human being" (see *Compendium on Medical Ethics*, 6th ed., edited by David M. Feldman and Fred Rosner [New York: Federation of Jewish Philanthropies of New York, 1984], 144–45).

39. McCormick, *Health and Medicine*, 8; Ashley and O'Rourke, *Health Care Ethics*, 38–46; National Conference of Catholic Bishops, "Directives," 451–53, and "Pastoral Letter."

40. Kelly, *Theological Basis for Health Care*, 43.

41. Zohar, 31. Maimonides criticizes people who see a contradiction between health care and pure faith in God. "According to their defective and silly fancy, if a person is hungry and seeks bread to eat—whereby he is undoubtedly healed from that great pain—should we say that he has failed to trust in God? 'What madmen!' is the proper retort to them. For just as I, at the time of eating, thank God for having provided me with something to relieve my hunger, to sustain my life and my strength—so should I thank Him for having provided a cure which heals my illness, when I use it" (Commentary to Mishnah *Pesaḥim* 4:6, trans. Zohar, 30).

42. *Summa Theologiae*, I-II, q. 94, a. 2, in Blackfriars edition, v. 28, trans. Thomas Gilby (New York: McGraw-Hill and London: Eyre and Spottiswoode, 1966), 63; Janssens, "Artificial Insemination," 8–9. See similarly GS, 23–32, in *Vatican Council II*, pp. 924–32 ; McCormick, *Health and Medicine*, 55–56; Ashley and O'Rourke, *Health Care Ethics*, 8–9, 167; Kelly, *Theological Basis for Health Care*, 53.

43. McCormick, *Health and Medicine*, 55.

44. Borowitz, *Exploring Jewish Ethics*, 70–83.

45. *Leviticus Rabbah* 4:6.

46. McCormick, *Health and Medicine*, 55.

47. See, e.g., Borowitz, *Exploring Jewish Ethics*, 19, 182–84; Dorff, *Matters of Life and Death*, 33; Newman, *Past Imperatives*, 154; and chapter 2 in this book. See also Jacob Neusner, "Was Rabbinic Judaism Really 'Ethnic'?" *Catholic Biblical Quarterly* 57 (1995): 281–305.

48. The literature exploring the ethics of the Noahide laws was very limited because until recent times virtually no non-Jews were interested in considering ethical insights emerging from the Jewish tradition.

49. Mishnah, *Gittin* 5:8; Talmud, *Gittin* 61a, *Sanhedrin* 105a; Maimonides, *Mishneh Torah*, "Laws of Idolatry" 10:5, "Laws of Gifts to the Poor" 7:7, "Laws of Mourning" 14:12, "Laws of Kings" 10:12; Louis Finkelstein, "Human Equality in the Jewish Tradition," in *Aspects of Equality*, ed. Lyman Bryson, Clarence H. Faust, Louis Finkelstein, and R. M. MacIver (New York: Harper and Brothers, 1956), 179–205. Finkelstein writes that although Judaism includes differing views over the form in which human existence will continue after death, "all agreed that immortality is open to everyone, if he chooses to follow the way of righteousness" (204).

50. Borowitz, *Exploring Jewish Ethics*, 99. See also Mishnah, *Sanhedrin* 4:5; Simon Greenberg, *A Jewish Philosophy and Pattern of Life* (New York: Jewish Theological Seminary of America, 1981), esp. 219–21.

51. See John Paul II, "Service Requesting Pardon," *Origins* 29 (2000): 645–48; International Theological Commission, "Memory and Reconciliation: The Church and the Faults of the Past," *Origins* 29 (2000): 625–44. John Noonan observes, "For a period of over 1,200 years, during much of which the Catholic Church was dominant in Europe, popes, bishops, theologians regularly and unanimously denied the religious liberty of heretics. . . . It was universally taught that the duty of a good ruler was to extirpate not only heresy but heretics" ("Development in Moral Doctrine," *Theological Studies* 54 [1993]: 667–68).

52. According to the Council of Florence, "no one who is outside the Catholic Church, not just pagans, but Jews, heretics, and schismatics, can

share in eternal life" (Mahoney, *The Making of Moral Theology,* 195). See Mahoney, 193–202.

53. *Nostra Aetate: Declaration on the Relation of the Church to Non-Christian Religion,* in *Vatican Council II,* 738–742; *Dignitatis Humanae: Declaration on Religious Liberty [DH],* in *Vatican Council II,* 799–812; *GS* 1, in *Vatican Council II,* 903; Mahoney, *The Making of Moral Theology,* 96–102.

54. National Conference of Catholic Bishops, *Economic Justice for All: Pastoral Letter on Catholic Social Teaching and the U.S. Economy* (Washington, D.C.: United States Catholic Conference, 1986); Aaron L. Mackler, "Judaism, Justice, and Access to Health Care," *Kennedy Institute of Ethics Journal* 1 (1991): 143–61.

55. Feldman, *Health and Medicine in the Jewish Tradition,* 55–78; *GS,* 47–52, in *Vatican Council II,* 949–57; Ashley and O'Rourke, *Health Care Ethics,* 204–12. An additional good of marriage in the Catholic tradition is its status as a sacrament; in Judaism, the ritual of marriage is known as *kiddushin,* "sanctification." In Judaism, procreation is understood to be a mitzvah for those who are able to have children; see Mishnah *Yevamot* 6:6; *Shulḥan Arukh, Even Ha'ezer* 1; Feldman, *Health and Medicine in the Jewish Tradition,* 69–71; Dorff, *Matters of Life and Death,* 39–42.

56. McCormick, *Health and Medicine,* 56–57.

57. Although diverse views may be found in each tradition, Jewish approaches tend to be more accepting of the use of reproductive technologies, as discussed in chapter 6. Unlike traditional Roman Catholicism, Judaism accepts divorce, regarding it as regrettable but in some cases the least bad alternative for a couple. Homosexuality has become an issue of intense controversy in each tradition; this complex issue is beyond the scope of this book.

58. *DH* 2, in *Vatican Council II,* 800. "The Council further declares that the right to religious freedom is based on the very dignity of the human person as known through the revealed word of God and by reason itself." See also *GS,* 16, in *Vatican Council II,* 916–17.

59. Borowitz, *Exploring Jewish Ethics;* David H. Ellenson, "How to Draw Guidance from a Heritage: Jewish Approaches to Mortal Choices," in *Contemporary Jewish Ethics and Morality,* 135–38; Avram I. Reisner, "Care for the Terminally Ill: Halakhic Concepts and Values," in *Life and Death Responsibilities in Jewish Biomedical Ethics,* 250–53; and the discussion in chapter 3.

60. Irving Greenberg, "Toward a Covenantal Ethics of Medicine," 142.

61. Ashley and O'Rourke, *Health Care Ethics,* 186–87.

62. Bleich, "Introduction," in *Jewish Bioethics,* xv.

63. Ashley and O'Rourke, *Health Care Ethics,* 182–86.

64. Seymour Siegel, "Healing and the Definition of Death," in *Biomedical Ethics in Perspective of Jewish Teaching and Tradition*, ed. Isaac Frank (Washington, D.C.: College of Jewish Studies of Greater Washington, 1980), 33; cited in James J. McCartney, "The Right to Die: Perspectives from the Catholic and Jewish Traditions," in *To Die or Not to Die? Cross-Disciplinary, Cultural, and Legal Perspectives on the Right to Choose Death*, ed. Arthur S. Berger and Joyce Berger (New York: Praeger, 1990), 20.

Chapter 1

Methodology in Roman Catholic Moral Theology

IN THE INTRODUCTION I PRESENT THE AGENDA OF THIS BOOK and sketch core ethical values that are central in each tradition. Vital as such foundational elements are, they represent only the beginning of the process of articulating norms and judgments in bioethics. These values must be concretized and specified to determine which actions and practices will enable their appropriate realization for individuals, institutions, and communities. Granted that responsible stewardship is an ethical value that should shape a religious perspective on the possible use of reproductive technologies, what does stewardship actually mean in this context?

Moreover, there may be tension among differing values in a particular situation. A Jew or Catholic caring for a dying patient would be well advised to act in a manner supportive of values such as life, health, respect for patient choices, love, compassion, spiritual growth, family, responsible stewardship, fair allocation of resources in the community, and respect for God's sovereignty. What if the implications of these values are unclear, however, or appear to point in different directions? Would a judgment that a given life-sustaining treatment be forgone represent an infringement on divine sovereignty, or would continuing to prolong life artificially really be the infringement? Would prolongation of life always represent a benefit to the patient? If not, what would be the criteria for judging that an extension of life is not beneficial? What if a family's choice for an incapacitated patient appears to health care professionals to be less compassionate than alternatives or to represent an unfair or unwise allocation of resources?[1]

In this chapter and the following chapter, I sketch Roman Catholic and Jewish methodologies in bioethics. First I present a brief overview of and orientation to ethical reasoning in each tradition. I devote attention to areas of dispute within each tradition, as well as to common tendencies. I also note general points of similarity and difference between the traditions. Catholic moral approaches are centered most commonly on natural law—representing reason and experience—along with magisterial teaching, though tradition represents an important source of moral knowledge. Jewish approaches generally are based on tradition, especially halakhah (Jewish law), although reason and experience have always been part of the process as well. Within each tradition, a spectrum of views may be found on the relationship between general ethical values, such as human well-being, and specific moral norms.

Introduction

Roman Catholic ethics is marked by themes of grace and love. For Catholics (and other Christians), the central manifestation of God's gracious love is Jesus Christ, the son of God and second person of the Trinity, who came to humanity for their salvation. God's love also permeates creation, created by God the Father and through Christ. By God's grace, humans are oriented toward community with God and other humans in God's kingdom. The Holy Spirit, the third person of the Trinity, is present in the "one holy catholic and apostolic Church," in the faith of its members, in its sacraments, and in its magisterial teaching.[2]

Roman Catholic morality concerns the actions, norms, and virtues appropriate to this faith. Moral theology emerged as a distinct discipline in the sixteenth century but has remained closely connected with other areas of theology and the life of faith generally. Moral theology has been defined as "that portion of the theological enterprise which attempts to discern the implications of revelation for human behavior, to answer the question: 'How ought we, who have been gifted by God, to live.'"[3] Traditional moral theology turns to a variety of sources of moral knowledge in addressing this question. These sources include Scripture, tradition, reason and experience, and the magisterial teaching authority of the Catholic Church.[4] All of these sources play vital roles in ethical deliberation. In the traditional Catholic understanding, these sources cannot fundamentally disagree because all ultimately reflect the same truth; accordingly, each source is properly understood in light of the others. Catholic thinkers have varying understandings of the meaning of and relative priority to be accorded to these sources.

Reason and Experience: Natural Law

Appeals to human reason and experience are frequent in classical and contemporary Roman Catholic ethics. Such appeals commonly are presented in terms of natural law. Such approaches attend to patterns of meaning found in creation and center on a normative model of human nature or the human person.

Natural law was defined by Thomas Aquinas as "the sharing in the Eternal law by intelligent creatures." For Thomas, all elements of God's creation are endowed by God with their proper ends or purposes, fulfillment of which represents their flourishing, in accord with the divinely prescribed order. Human ends include self-preservation, procreation and education of children, communal life, and knowledge of and communion with God. Whereas most creatures follow their natural inclinations without thought, humans are able to use reason to discern good and evil. They are called on to choose the path that God in wisdom and providence has laid out for human fulfillment and well-being in the structure of creation.[5]

Historicity

Catholic thinkers differ with regard to several issues related to natural law, including the extent to which the normative model of human good is constant or changing across cultures and in history; the elements of human well-being to be included in the normative model; and the extent to which natural law supports exceptionless moral norms (including the significance of the principle of double effect). Historically, classical approaches tended to exhibit an essentialist, static view of human nature. Accordingly, moral norms, at least at a basic or general level, could apply universally to all humans.[6] Moral norms remain unchanged through history. As expressed by Henry Davis in 1935, "A writer on Moral Theology today must be indebted beyond measure to the labour of past writers, for the matter is one that has been treated with the greatest acumen and scholarship during well-nigh three centuries, and *there is no room for originality.*"[7] Especially over the past half-century, moral theologians increasingly have come to regard nature and humanity as dynamic, subject to significant historical change. Indeed, the Second Vatican Council, in *Gaudium et Spes*, suggested that in contemporary times "the human race has passed from a rather static concept of reality to a more dynamic, evolutionary one."[8]

Few contemporary thinkers advocate either a completely static and unchanging understanding of humanity or the opposite extreme of a thoroughgoing historical relativism. Within the broad middle ground, some thinkers emphasize the dynamic openness of morality. For example, Richard McCormick presents natural law as a "dynamically inviting possibility."[9] Louis Janssens argues that "new possibilities . . . should not be gratuitously accepted simply because they are new, but neither should we rashly reject them." Janssens adds, "Ethics is fundamentally a way of living and in its own growth must keep step with human life itself as it unfolds through history. That is precisely what we mean when we say that it must be dynamic, as human life itself which it directs and leads."[10]

Other theologians—who similarly claim a middle ground—place greater emphasis on what they consider unchanging in humanity and ethics. Benedict Ashley and Kevin O'Rourke assert that "historicity itself implies continuity, identity, and community. . . . Therefore human persons all have some basic common needs that characterize them as humans. . . . Keeping in mind this delicate balance between the universality and permanence of human nature on the one hand and its historicity and cultural variation on the other, Christians seek moral standards that are transcultural yet sensitive to existential realities." This approach emphasizes the unchanging and essentially human, while acknowledging but according less significance to historical change.[11]

Significance of the Physical and Biological

A related issue involves the normative significance of the (relatively unchanging) physical and biological aspects of humanity. Classical moral theology understood biological teleology as central to natural law. Indeed, for Thomas Aquinas the biological capacities that humans share with animals can be even more strongly normative than interpersonal ethical norms. "The plan of nature comes from God, and therefore a violation of this plan, as by unnatural sins, is an affront to God, the ordainer of nature."[12]

This powerful commitment to biological teleology continued through modern times. In 1946 Francis X. Hürth wrote, "Human beings only have disposal of the use of their organs and their faculties with respect to the end which the Creator, in his formation of them, has intended. This end for humans then is both the biological law and the moral law, such that the latter obliges them to live according to the biological law."[13]

Critics characterize such approaches as "physicalism," which considers "man in terms of distinct faculties, each created by God with a particular goal or purpose, defined in terms of the physical structure of the faculty."[14] In their view, physicalism is inappropriately narrow in focus, slighting crucial aspects of the human and of human flourishing. The normative standard should not be human nature or the human organism but "the human person integrally and adequately considered."[15] Thinkers who advocate a broader personalism acknowledge that physical and biological aspects of the person have some significance; "the person is a subject in corporeality," and "our body forms a part of the integrated subject that we are; corporeal and spiritual."[16] Nevertheless, in cases of conflict between biological and other elements, decisive weight is accorded to more broadly personal, spiritual, and social concerns.[17]

Other contemporary theologians generally acknowledge the significance of broad personal concerns but claim that biological patterns of reality remain crucial in defining the human person and human flourishing. Spiritual and social values appropriately are pursued as part of the human good but not in ways that violate the physical norms that also constitute the human good. According to Ashley and O'Rourke, in cases of conflict physical and biological concerns may be decisive:

> All human acts, however spiritual, are also acts of the body, as the Jewish tradition has always taught. Consequently, for an act to be

truly human, it must respect the inherent teleology or normal biological functions of the body and its organs, not because these are
superior to other dimensions of the person, but because their functions are not merely animal but truly human and absolutely necessary to think, love, and act as human beings.[18]

Exceptionless Norms and Double Effect

Along with disputes about the significance of historical change and
biological patterns go divergent understandings of the types of moral
norms that can be exceptionless and the principle of double effect. As
classically understood, this principle recognizes as morally valid some
actions that directly cause a good effect while indirectly causing an evil
effect. For example, a hysterectomy may be performed for a pregnant
woman with cancer of the uterus, intentionally and directly removing
cancerous tissue and saving the woman's life, though it indirectly and
unintentionally causes the death of the unborn child. Intentionally and
directly taking the life of the unborn child, however, would be
regarded as absolutely forbidden, even in an unusual case in which this
action would be required to save the woman's life. As laid out by Gerald Kelly, the principle prescribes that an action that causes both good
and evil effects may be performed if, and only if, all four of the following conditions are fulfilled:

1. The action, considered by itself and independently of its effects,
   must not be morally evil. . . .
2. The evil effect must not be the means of producing the good
   effect. . . . The evil effects . . . are simply unavoidable by-prod-
   ucts of [actions] designed to produce the good effects . . .
3. The evil effect is sincerely not intended, but merely tolerated.
4. There must be a proportionate reason for performing the action,
   in spite of its evil consequence. . . . According to a sound prudential estimate, the good to be obtained is of sufficient value to
   compensate for the evil that must be tolerated.[19]

Advocates of the principle of double effect suggest that this
approach allows for action despite ambiguous circumstances (and
thus avoids a paralyzing "moral purism"), while respecting the

absolute norms of objective morality. Some actions (such as intentional and direct killing of the innocent, masturbation, and artificial contraception) are intrinsically evil and may never be performed, even when they would appear to produce beneficial consequences.[20]

Other theologians—often termed proportionalists—would focus almost exclusively on the third and fourth clauses of the principle of double effect as formulated above, concerning intentions and consequences (proportionality). They argue that "for Thomas and for today's moralists the *finis operis* (the end of the act-in-itself) can never be specified apart from the *finis operantis* (the intention of the agent, or the end of the total human act)."[21] For example, traditionalists would claim that masturbation to obtain a sperm sample for medical testing would fail by the principle of double effect because an intrinsically evil act (masturbation) would be the means to achieve the end of medical testing that could yield useful knowledge. Proportionalists would claim that the act involved cannot be fully specified without taking into account the beneficial consequences of testing and the intention of the man involved to help him and his wife have a child. It is not simply an act of masturbation that happens to lead to an extrinsic positive consequence; the consequences and intentionality affect the definition of the act itself. Many proportionalists would acknowledge the occurrence of orgasm outside of marital intercourse as an ontic or premoral evil, which should not be intentionally sought and would count against the acceptability of the action. Such ontic evil would be acceptable only in the context of an action that achieved enough good to outweigh this cost and in which the ontic evil was unavoidable.[22]

Most proportionalists, then, would agree with traditionalists that biological teleology bears some normative weight. They would argue, however, that biological teleology cannot be decisive in itself, partly because of the weight accorded to personal and spiritual goods and partly because of greater flexibility in connection with the principle of double effect. Similarly, proportionalists would acknowledge that some acts could be intrinsically evil, but they would argue that intrinsically evil acts cannot be defined a priori, on the basis solely of the act itself, narrowly construed. Intrinsically evil acts may be identified only a posteriori, with attention to consequences and intentions. For example, "abortion for convenience" might be intrinsically evil and never permissible; but "abortion" (or "direct killing of an unborn child") might be justifiable under unusual circumstances.[23]

Scripture and Tradition

The Catholic Bible includes both the New Testament and the Old Testament, including deuterocanonical or "apochryphal" books such as Tobit and Ecclesiasticus.[24] Moral theologians of diverse views support, in principle, a crucial role for the Bible in moral life and reflection. Few theologians would disagree with the proclamation of Vatican II that the study of Scripture "should be the very soul of sacred theology." "All the preaching of the Church, as indeed the entire Christian religion, should be nourished and ruled by sacred Scripture."[25] Many theologians would endorse the counsel of Vatican II that moral theology in particular "should draw more fully on the teaching of holy Scripture."[26]

At the same time, detailed analysis of Scripture generally receives relatively little attention in the formulation of specific ethical judgments.[27] In part this focus on other sources of moral knowledge reflects a sense that Scripture will not offer precise guidance for complex contemporary challenges. In general, a biblical text may allow for several different interpretations because "in sacred Scripture, God speaks through men in human fashion." Properly interpreting the Bible requires formulating judgments in light of the historical and literary context of the human authors.[28] Extrapolating from the biblical teaching to contemporary challenges is even more complex. McCormick argues that although Scripture is essential to human morality, it should not be expected to yield precise answers to concrete contemporary issues. Such an expectation would be "a form of medical-moral fundamentalism that would use Scripture as a kind of 'truth cabinet,' finding answers there to questions about which the sacred writers were totally ignorant." Instead, although "the sources of faith do enlighten such problems," they do so indirectly. "Scripture nourishes our overall perspectives, telling us through Christ the kinds of people we ought to be and become, and the type of world we ought to create. It does not give us concrete answers to tragic conflict cases or relieve us of the messy and arduous work of search, deliberation, and discussion."[29]

Where the guidance of Scripture is unambiguous, there may be little need for detailed analysis. Writings in fields such as bioethics focus on areas in which Scripture is not decisive and underdetermines the result; in these cases it is supplemented by reason, tradition, and the magisterium, which assist in the fine-tuning of moral judgment. Because of the basic agreement of the sources of moral knowledge, one may readily turn from one to another, so a theologian may focus on a natural law analysis (or magisterial pronouncements) when the guidance of Scripture is inconclusive.[30] Reason in general, and natural law in particular, are regarded as supported both by general theological understandings and by Scripture itself.[31] Accordingly, a moral theologian investigating complex biomedical challenges must remain mindful of biblical injunctions of love and faith but may focus his or her writings on the details of scientific facts, the significance of basic human goods, and the relevance of reasonable moral norms.

Moreover, in the Catholic tradition Scripture is read not as an independent document (or, at least, not only as such) but through the eyes of the present and historical community. Tradition both conveys and complements the written Scripture. According to *Dei Verbum*, "Sacred Tradition and sacred Scripture, then, are bound closely together, and communicate one with the other. For both of them, flowing out from the same divine well-spring, come together." "Sacred Tradition and sacred Scripture make up a single sacred deposit of the Word of God, which is entrusted to the Church." In addition, the magisterium's interpretation will provide a clearer statement of the significance of Scripture for a given issue than would the unvarnished Scriptural text itself. "The task of giving an authentic interpretation of the Word of God, whether in its written form or in the form of Tradition, has been entrusted to the living teaching office of the Church alone."[32]

Tradition is widely recognized to include elements of development as well as constancy. Pope John Paul II acknowledges that "this truth of the moral law—like that of the 'deposit of faith'—unfolds down the centuries."[33] McCormick writes that "tradition, in its best theological sense, refers to a living reality. . . . A living tradition includes the formative effects of the past. It is instructed by the past, but . . . not paralyzed by it." Past formulations are necessarily limited; the community is always in the process of seeking to improve or "purify" the living tradition.[34] Different authors differ somewhat on the extent to which past sources of the tradition are decisive. In practice, this question tends to be subordinate to the question of authority: the extent to which the central magisterium determines which positions are consistent with natural law and the authentic interpretation of the tradition, as well as the extent to which individual theologians (or others) may support a position on the basis of reasoned argument and conscience.

Authority and the Magisterium

Most Catholic theologians acknowledge that significant authority is held both by church officials and by individuals forming their own consciences. Theologians differ in their understandings of the precise nature of and relative strength of these different sources of authority. Each individual priest represents an important source of authority, in preaching and teaching generally and in the context of evaluating actions in the sacrament of Penance and Reconciliation in particular. In this sacrament, the penitent confesses his or her sins to the priest, who determines the appropriate penance and offers sacramental absolution that represents God's forgiveness. Classically, this exchange is likened to the healing offered to a patient by a physician or "like an act of judgment by which sentence is pronounced on him by a judge."[35]

Although the priest represents a proximate authority in evaluating particular actions, an ultimate authority is represented by the church's central teaching authority—the magisterium. Moral theologians generally recognize an important role for the magisterium but differ about the extent of the role and, in particular, the legitimacy of a theologian holding a view (typically based on natural law justification) that differs from that of official church teaching. The word "magisterium" literally means "mastery" and refers to the authority of the master. In the Middle Ages the word referred to the mastery of the teacher, including both the professor in the university and the bishop. By the First Vatican Council of 1870, the term had come to refer to the centralized teaching authority of the church hierarchy, headed by the Pope.[36]

The basis for magisterial authority is that it traditionally is understood as safeguarding the "deposit of faith." This "sacred deposit" was entrusted by God to the Church, and "the task of giving an authentic interpretation . . . has been entrusted to the living teaching office of the Church alone." Those who exercise the magisterium are not understood simply to have been given power to make decisions as they see fit. Instead, the magisterium "teaches only what has been handed down to it. At the divine command and with the help of the Holy Spirit, it listens to this devotedly, guards it with dedication and expounds it faithfully. All that it proposes for belief as being divinely revealed is drawn from this single deposit of faith."[37] Accordingly, a crucial source of moral knowledge is provided by the "constant guidance of Jesus through his Church and its authority to teach."[38]

Vatican II acknowledges that at the current time the Catholic Church is still a "pilgrim Church," that is not (yet) perfect and "does not always have a ready answer to every question."[39] At the same time, it expresses confidence that "the whole body of the faithful . . . cannot err in matters of belief. This characteristic is shown in the supernatural appreciation of the faith (*sensus fidei*) of the whole people, when, 'from the bishops to the last of the faithful,' they manifest a universal consent in matters of faith and morals. By this appreciation of the faith, aroused and sustained by the Spirit of truth, the People of God, guided by the sacred teaching authority (*magisterium*), and obeying it, receives not the mere word of men, but truly the word of God."[40] To maintain shared loyalty to the truth as understood by the Church, the faithful "are obliged to submit to their bishops' decision, made in the name of Christ, in matters of faith and morals, and to adhere to it with a ready and respectful allegiance of mind. This loyal submission of the will and intellect must be given, in a special way, to the authentic teaching authority of the Roman Pontiff." When the bishops acting collectively—as in an ecumenical council—"are in agreement that a particular teaching is to be held definitively and absolutely," these "decisions must be adhered to with the loyal and obedient assent of faith."[41]

For some theologians, the appropriate response of the faithful to magisterial teaching is simply acceptance and obedience. A classic expression of this view was offered by Pope Pius XII in his encyclical *Humani Generis*. The ordinary teaching of the church is supported by

Jesus's assurance to the disciples, "He who heareth you, heareth Me." "If the Supreme Pontiffs in their official documents purposely pass judgment on a matter up to that time under dispute, it is obvious that the matter, according to the mind and will of the same Pontiffs, cannot be any longer considered a question open to discussion among theologians." "The most noble office of theology is to show how a doctrine defined by the Church is contained in the sources of Revelation . . . in that sense in which it has been defined by the Church."[42]

Other theologians suggest that although magisterial teaching represents an important source of moral knowledge and deserves significant deference, it does not automatically trump other sources of moral knowledge that also are recognized as legitimate. For McCormick, magisterial teaching should be heard with "a docility of mind and will, . . . a desire to assimilate the teaching," and "a readiness to reassess one's own position in light of the teaching." Yet although such docility always entails respect, it does not always necessitate agreement and obedience.[43]

The possibility that individuals may differ from magisterial teaching is supported by the authority of conscience—also strongly asserted by Vatican II. "Deep within his conscience man discovers a law which he must obey. . . . His dignity lies in observing this law, and by it he will be judged." To be sure, "in forming their consciences the faithful must pay careful attention to the sacred and certain teaching of the Church." Yet "it is through his conscience that man sees and recognizes the demands of the divine law. He is bound to follow this conscience faithfully in all his activity. . . . Therefore he must not be forced to act contrary to his conscience."[44] Accordingly, James Hanigan presents conscience as "the ultimate, subjective norm of morality." "Consequently, while it is not enough not to see what is wrong or right about a practice in order to have grounds for a conscientious dissent, for the individual who sees—or is sincerely convinced that he or she sees—that the truth about the good lies elsewhere than authority proclaims, conscientious dissent is not only a possibility; it is an obligation."[45]

Theologians who argue against too decisive a role for the magisterium also express concern not to undermine the natural law basis of Catholic morality. David Kelly warns of a *de facto* "ecclesiastical positivism," in which morality is determined on the basis of what church authority has posited rather than on what actually promotes the human good. "Since such decrees are now seen as *de facto* necessary for an understanding of the (supposedly natural) moral law, the natural law becomes natural only theoretically," Kelly writes. "In practice, it is derived from the (supernaturally guaranteed) teachings of the Roman Catholic Church."[46]

Conclusion

Roman Catholic moral theologians agree on the importance of several sources of moral knowledge. Human reason and experience, understood in terms of natural law, tends to be the source that receives greatest attention. Theologians express varying views about the significance of historical change and biological patterns of meaning and about the possibility and characteristics of exceptionless moral norms. Controversies also may be found with respect to authority—especially the extent to which the pronouncements of the central magisterium are decisive and the extent to which individuals may conscientiously dissent on the basis of other sources of knowledge. Scripture and tradition are honored and help to provide the framing context in which debates about natural law and authority are formulated but tend not to be central in methodological debates or in the formulation of particular norms and judgments. As chapter 2 notes, Jewish thinkers recognize similar sources of moral knowledge and, like their Catholic colleagues, engage in methodological debates. In Judaism, however, tradition plays a more central role, both in disputes about methodology and in concrete applications.

Notes

1. See Aaron L. Mackler, "Cases and Principles in Jewish Bioethics: Toward a Holistic Model," in *Contemporary Jewish Ethics and Morality: A Reader*, ed. Elliot N. Dorff and Louis E. Newman (New York: Oxford University Press, 1995), 182.

2. See *Catechism of the Catholic Church* (Mission Hills, Calif.: Benziger, 1994), including the Nicene Creed, pp. 49–50.

3. Timothy E. O'Connell, *Principles for a Catholic Morality*, rev. ed. (New York: HarperSanFrancisco, HarperCollins, 1990), 7. See also ibid., 18–19; Bernard Häring, *The Law of Christ*, vol. 1, trans. Edwin G. Kaiser (Westminster, Md.: Newman, 1963), 17–20.

4. E.g., Charles E. Curran, *The Catholic Moral Tradition Today: A Synthesis* (Washington, D.C.: Georgetown University Press, 1999), 47–55; James P. Hanigan, *As I Have Loved You: The Challenge of Christian Ethics* (Mahwah, N.J.: Paulist, 1986), 19.

5. Thomas Aquinas, *Summa Theologiae* I-II q. 91, a. 1–2; q. 94, a. 2; in Blackfriars ed., vol. 28, trans. Thomas Gilby (New York: McGraw-Hill and London: Eyre and Spottiswoode, 1966), 19–25, 77–83. As this passage is paraphrased by Pope John Paul II, "In order to perfect himself in his specific order, the person must do good and avoid evil, be concerned for the transmission and preservation of life, refine and develop the riches of the material world, cultivate social life, seek truth, practice good, and contemplate beauty"; *Veritatis Splendor: The Splendor of Truth [VS]* (Washington, D.C.: United States Catholic Conference, 1993), n. 51, p. 80. John Mahoney offers this summary of classical natural law theory: "Man as a rational being sharing in God's providential activity is aware of what God has impressed in his nature and he is capable of freely accepting and embracing the order of his being and his place in the divine scheme of things. This knowing and free acceptance of his nature as created and destined by God is man's observance of the law of his nature, or of the 'natural law'" (*The Making of Moral Theology: A Study of the Roman Catholic Tradition* [New York: Clarendon Press, Oxford University Press, 1987], 78). Similarly, for Benedict M. Ashley and Kevin D. O'Rourke, "Human beings act morally when they live in such a way as to satisfy in a consistent and harmonious way those needs basic to human life and common to all human beings. Thus the natural law is our human sharing in God's own wisdom about what kind of living will best fulfill the nature which the Creator has given us by creating us as bodily beings who also in our spiritual intelligence and free will image God" (*Health Care Ethics: A Theological Analysis*, 4th ed. [Washington, D.C.: Georgetown University Press, 1997], 156–57).

6. Though Thomas Aquinas noted that "in questions of action, however, practical truth and goodwill are not the same for everybody with respect to particular decisions" (*Summa Theologiae* I-II q. 94, a. 5; Blackfriars ed., vol. 28, p. 89).

7. Henry Davis, *Moral and Pastoral Theology,* vol. 1 (New York: Sheed and Ward, 1935), vii; emphasis added.

8. *Gaudium et Spes: Pastoral Constitution on the Church in the Modern World [GS]*, n. 5, in *The Documents of Vatican II*, ed. Walter M. Abbott (New York: Corpus, 1966), 204.

9. Richard A. McCormick, "Human Significance and Christian Significance," in *Norm and Context in Christian Ethics*, ed. Gene H. Outka and Paul Ramsey (New York: Charles Scribner's Sons, 1968), 239, quoting Louis Monden, *Sin, Liberty and Law* (New York: Sheed and Ward, 1965), 89. See also Richard McCormick, *Health and Medicine in the Catholic Tradition* (New York: Crossroad, 1987), 17. For David F. Kelly, "natural law theory is the claim that human persons discover right and wrong by their God-given reason and life experience, examining individually and collectively the patterns of creation *as God is creating it*" (*Critical Care Ethics: Treatment Decisions in American Hospitals* [St. Louis: Sheed and Ward, 1991], 85; emphasis added).

10. Louis Janssens, "Artificial Insemination: Ethical Considerations," *Louvain Studies* 7 (1980): 11.

11. Ashley and O'Rourke, *Health Care Ethics*, 172–73. Ashley and O'Rourke present themselves as following "the classical methodology of moral judgment . . . to which we add more attention to human historicity and subjectivity in our understanding of human needs and the means available to satisfy them" (173). Pope John Paul II discusses "permanent structural elements of man" and presents central moral norms as unchanging and immutable. He allows some—though relatively modest—significance for historical change. "There is a need to seek out and to discover the most adequate formulation for universal and permanent moral norms in the light of different cultural contexts, a formulation most capable of ceaselessly expressing their historical relevance. . . . This truth of the moral law . . . unfolds down the centuries: the norms expressing the truth remain valid in their substance, but must be specified and determined '*eodem sensu eademque sententia*' in the light of historical circumstances." This determination is to be carried out by the church's magisterium, as discussed below (*VS*, nn. 51–53, 115; pp. 79–85, 172).

12. *Summa Theologiae* II-II, 154, 11–12, in Blackfriars ed., vol. 43, trans. Thomas Gilby (New York: McGraw-Hill and London: Eyre and Spottiswoode, 1968), pp. 247–49. Accordingly, "unnatural vice" (masturbation, homosexuality, or bestiality) is a graver sin than rape or incest (despite the harm that these sins entail for human persons) or sacrilege. "We have contended that sins against nature are sins against God. And they are graver than the depravity of sacrilege to the extent that the order of nature is more basic and stable than the order of reason we build on it."

13. Francis X. Hürth, "La Fécondation Artificielle," *Nouvelle Révue Théologique* 68 (1946): 416; translation in McCormick, *Health and Medicine*, 19.

14. David F. Kelly, *The Emergence of Roman Catholic Medical Ethics in North America* (New York: Mellen, 1979), 245. See also Charles E. Curran,

Contemporary Problems in Moral Theology (Notre Dame, Ind.: Fides, 1970), esp. 104–42.

15. McCormick, *Health and Medicine*, 15, citing an official commentary on *GS* 51, which sets forth a standard of "the nature of the human person and his acts" (in *Documents of Vatican II*, 256).

16. Janssens, "Artificial Insemination," 5. See also *GS*, n. 14, in *Vatican Council II: The Conciliar and Post Conciliar Documents*, new rev. ed., ed. Austin Flannery (Northport, N.Y.: Costello, 1996), 914–15; McCormick, *Health and Medicine*, 16.

17. Kelly, *Emergence of Roman Catholic Medical Ethics*, 419. "In general, personalism refers to that modality of application of theological principles whereby an emphasis is placed on the entire personal complexus of the act in its human dimensions, circumstances, and consequences. In contradistinction to the modalities which preceded it, personalism does not limit its scope to the physical or biological qualities of the action, but rather extends its purview to psychological, social, and spiritual dimensions." Charles E. Curran similarly writes, "The physical is part of the human but only one part, and the total human can never be reduced only to the physical. The human is made up of many dimensions" (*Catholic Moral Tradition Today*, 155).

18. Ashley and O'Rourke, *Health Care Ethics*, 173. See also John Paul II, *VS*, n. 48, pp. 75–76. According to the Congregation for the Doctrine of the Faith:

> It is only in keeping with his true nature that the human person can achieve self-realization as a "unified totality": and this nature is at the same time corporal and spiritual. By virtue of its substantial union with a spiritual soul, the human body cannot be considered as a mere complex of tissues, organs and functions, nor can it be evaluated in the same way as the body of animals; rather it is a constitutive part of the person who manifests and expresses himself through it. The natural moral law expresses and lays down the purposes, rights and duties which are based upon the bodily and spiritual nature of the human person. Therefore this law cannot be thought of as simply a set of norms on the biological level; rather it must be defined as the rational order whereby man is called by the Creator to direct and regulate his life and actions and in particular to make use of his own body (*Donum Vitae: Instruction on Respect for Human Life in Its Origin and on the Dignity of Procreation* [Washington, D.C.: United States Catholic Conference, 1987], 8).

19. Gerald Kelly, *Medico-Moral Problems* (St. Louis: Catholic Health Association, 1958), 12–14.

20. Ashley and O'Rourke, *Health Care Ethics,* 191–93; *VS,* nn. 71–83, pp. 108–27.

21. Kelly, *Emergence of Roman Catholic Medical Ethics,* 253n.

22. Part of the debate involves interpretation of the classic passage from Thomas Aquinas that provides a source of the principle of double effect. According to Aquinas, "An act of self-defense may have two effects: the saving of one's life, and the killing of the attacker. Now such an act of self-defense is not illegitimate just because the agent intends to save his own life. . . . An act that is properly motivated may, nevertheless, become vitiated if it is not proportionate to the end intended. And this is why somebody who uses more violence than is necessary to defend himself will be doing something wrong"; *Summa Theologiae* II-II, q. 64, a. 7; in Blackfriars ed., vol. 38, trans. Marcus Lefébure (New York: McGraw-Hill and London: Eyre and Spottiswoode, 1975), 43. Some traditionalists would interpret this passage in accord with the four conditions noted above: The striking of the aggressor has the good effect of stopping the assault and the bad effect, not strictly intended, of killing the aggressor. For proportionalists, the death of the aggressor represents ontic evil that may be justified to the extent that it is necessary to save one's life. See Kelly, *Emergence of Roman Catholic Medical Ethics,* 254–55; Peter Knauer, "The Hermeneutic Function of the Principle of Double Effect," in *Readings in Moral Theology No. 1: Moral Norms and Catholic Tradition,* ed. Charles E. Curran and Richard A. McCormick (New York: Paulist, 1979), 1–39.

23. Kelly, *Emergence of Roman Catholic Medical Ethics,* 251–58; Richard McCormick, "Some Early Reactions to *Veritatis Splendor,*" *Theological Studies* 55 (1994): 495–99, 503–4; Anthony Kosnik et al., *Human Sexuality: New Directions in American Catholic Thought* (New York: Paulist, 1977), 227; Ashley and O'Rourke, *Health Care Ethics,* 159–64.

24. Within Scripture, the four Gospels are accorded a "special place" (*Dei Verbum: Dogmatic Constitution on Divine Revelation [DV],* n. 18, in *Vatican Council II,* p. 760).

25. *DV,* nn. 24, 21; *Optatam Totius: Decree on the Training of Priests [OT],* n. 16; in *Vatican Council II,* pp. 764, 762, 719.

26. *OT,* n.16, in *Vatican Council II,* p. 720.

27. James F. Gustafson observes that for Roman Catholic ethics from Trent until Vatican II, "the role of Scripture was frequently one of citation of texts that supported natural law arguments" (*Protestant and Roman Catholic Ethics: Prospects for Rapprochement* [Chicago: University of Chicago Press, 1978], 96). Although the situation has become more nuanced, at least in the

writings of many theologians, Scripture tends not to be at the forefront of bioethical writings as much as natural law, tradition, or magisterial pronouncements.

28. DV, n. 12, in Vatican Council II, p. 757.

29. McCormick, Health and Medicine, 47–48. See similarly Curran, Catholic Moral Tradition Today, 48–52.

30. As Gustafson observes, for Catholic moral theology Scripture dovetails neatly with natural law arguments. "There are no serious cleavages between the revealed moral will of God and the natural moral law, as both have the same ultimate source" (Protestant and Roman Catholic Ethics, 26).

31. See Gustafson, Protestant and Roman Catholic Ethics, 100–11; Josef Fuchs, Natural Law: A Theological Investigation, trans. Helmut Reckter and John A. Dowling (New York: Sheed and Ward, 1965), 14–32.

32. DV, nn. 8–12, in Vatican Council II, pp. 754–57. "It is clear, therefore, that, in the supremely wise arrangement of God, sacred Tradition, sacred Scripture and the Magisterium of the Church are so connected that one of them cannot stand without the others" (DV, n. 10, in Vatican Council II, p. 756).

33. VS, n. 53, p. 85. John Paul II specifies that the determination of appropriate development is made by the magisterium, "preceded and accompanied by" the thought of believers and theologians.

34. McCormick, Health and Medicine, 3–4.

35. Mahoney, The Making of Moral Theology, 24, quoting the Council of Trent, and generally 1–36; Catechism of the Catholic Church, 357–74. Vatican II qualifies this traditional stance: "For guidance and spiritual strength, let them [laypersons] turn to the clergy; but let them realize that their pastors will not always be so expert as to have a ready answer to every problem (even every grave problem) that arises; this is not the role of the clergy: it is rather up to the laymen to shoulder their responsibilities under the guidance of Christian wisdom and with eager attention to the teaching authority of the Church" (GS, 43, in Vatican Council II, 944). The priest also exercises authority in particular cases when he makes dispensations.

36. Francis A. Sullivan, Magisterium: Teaching Authority in the Catholic Church (New York: Paulist, 1983), 24–26; Mahoney, The Making of Moral Theology, 116–20.

37. DV, n. 10, in Vatican Council II, p. 755–56.

38. Ashley and O'Rourke, Health Care Ethics, 183.

39. Lumen Gentium: Dogmatic Constitution on the Church [LG], n. 48; GS, n. 33; in Vatican Council II, 407–8, 933.

40. LG, n. 12, in Vatican Council II, 363.

41. LG, n. 25, in Vatican Council II, 379–80.

42. Pius XII, *Humani Generis*, nn. 29, 36 (New York: Paulist, 1950), pp. 11–12, citing Luke 10:16. More recently, the Congregation for the Doctrine of the Faith has urged, "When the magisterium proposes 'in a definitive way' truths concerning faith and morals, which even if not divinely revealed are nevertheless strictly and intimately connected with revelation, these must be firmly accepted and held. When the magisterium, not intending to act 'definitively,' teaches a doctrine to aid a better understanding of revelation and make explicit its contents, or to recall how some teaching is in conformity with the truths of faith or finally to guard against ideas that are incompatible with these truths, the response called for is that of the religious submission of will and intellect" ("The Ecclesial Vocation of the Theologian," n. 23, *Origins* 20 [1990]: 122).

43. McCormick, *Health and Medicine*, 69–70.

44. GS, 16, *Dignitatis Humanae: Declaration on Religious Liberty*, nn. 14, 3; in *Vatican Council II*, 916, 811, 801. See also *Catechism of the Catholic Church*, nn. 1776–1802, pp. 438–42.

45. Hanigan, *As I Have Loved You*, 142.

46. David F. Kelly, *Emergence of Roman Catholic Medical Ethics*, 365, and generally 311–401, 429–36. David Kelly responds in part to the attempts of Gerald Kelly to harmonize the sources of authority. Gerald Kelly claims that Catholic moralists have a high degree of expertise in the objective "science of ethics." In addition, the church has teaching authority, granted by Christ, that includes authority in all aspects of divine revelation, understood to include natural law. "The Church not only claims divine authorization to interpret the moral law; it also claims that its teaching is a practical necessity for a clear and adequate knowledge of the law" (Gerald Kelly, *Medico-Moral Problems*, 31–34; similarly, 150–53).

Chapter 2

Methodology in Jewish Ethics

ETHICAL CONCERNS HAVE ALWAYS BEEN CENTRAL TO JUDAISM, and such concerns have been understood within the broad context of Jewish life. Basic concepts in Judaism include God; Torah, or "Teaching"; and the community of Israel, the Jewish people.[1] For Jews and Jewish thinkers across a wide spectrum of beliefs, individuals and the Jewish community as a whole participate in a covenantal relationship with God. Torah is central to this relationship and basic to Jewish life. God gave the Torah in love to the Jewish people—and through them to the world. In its narrowest sense, Torah refers to the first five books of the Bible: Genesis through Deuteronomy, traditionally termed the "Written Torah." More broadly, Torah includes the extensive "Oral Torah" and refers to all Jewish traditional teaching—in fact, all authentic Jewish thought and practice.[2]

Jewish ethics has been understood within this context, not sharply distinguished from other spheres of life. Indeed, Judaism has no distinct discipline analogous to Catholic moral theology. One example of this holistic approach may be found in the Holiness Code of the Book of Leviticus. This passage proclaims numerous ethical responsibilities, including the mandate to "love your neighbor as yourself," intermixed with ritual commandments. All represent aspects of the general injunction of this section: "You shall be holy, for I, the Lord your God am holy."[3] Both ethical and ritual perspectives are important in answering the question, "What ought I do?" For this code, as for the Jewish tradition in general, all aspects of human activity meld together holistically in a life of service to God and one's fellow.

Two additional features of the Holiness Code represent views that have been present throughout Judaism's development. First, the passage is introduced by an instruction from God to Moses: "Speak to the whole

Israelite community, and say to them . . ." (Lev. 19:2). The call to holiness, and all that follows, is understood not as pertaining exclusively or even primarily to individuals but to an entire community. Second, the commitment to holiness entails particular behavioral norms that are expected of individuals and the community. Such norms are traditionally termed mitzvot (singular: mitzvah, "commandment"). A mitzvah is a shared normative practice, expressing what members of the Jewish community may expect from one another. In the words of Abraham Heschel, "a mitzvah is an act which God and man have in common."[4]

Each mitzvah contributes to a system of halakhah, which literally means "path" or "way" and signifies Jewish law. Supporters argue that halakhah's role as a legal system provides for cohesion and a sense of community among Jews worldwide, as well as within local communities. It offers continuity with the past, maintaining continuity of the covenantal community over time and affording contemporary individuals the benefit of accumulated wisdom of the past. Halakhah traditionally has been understood to express both God's will and God's wise and beneficent counsel. Thus, it provides a means for the expression of God's love and of the Jew's love for God. Finally, the very fact of the centrality of halakhah to Jewish ethics over the millennia might be regarded as itself carrying normative weight. A halakhically centered approach simply is the Jewish way to do ethics; to use Wittgenstein's image, such are the rules of the language game of Jewish ethics.[5]

Although halakhah has been central to Jewish life and thought, it never has been exclusive. Accompanying halakhah has been aggadah, or narrative. This term broadly refers to Jewish theological reflection, lore, articulation of values, expressions of meaning, and cultivation of virtues. Returning to the Holiness Code of Leviticus 19, Moses Nahmanides (fourteenth century) writes that the opening call to holiness is not merely a classificatory heading but an injunction in its own right. Without this injunction, a person might observe all the rules yet be "a scoundrel with Torah license."[6] The call to holiness includes—but also goes beyond—the specific norms of halakhah. Classically, the relationship between halakhah and aggadah, between the letter and spirit of the law, is symbiotic.[7] In Heschel's image, halakhah is like a body, whereas aggadah is spirit. Halakhah without aggadah, its animating spirit, is like a corpse. Aggadah without halakhah, its worldly concretization, is like a ghost, too ethereal to be realized.[8] The specification of halakhah and aggadah and the relative priority of each when they appear to conflict are central issues of dispute in contemporary Jewish thought.

Reason and Experience

All Jewish thinkers acknowledge a role for reason and experience in shaping ethics. Understandings of this role and its relation to tradition vary widely. In classical Judaism, appeals to universal reason and human experience are less central than are appeals to sacred texts and tradition. At the same time, Judaism has considered all of humanity to be participating in a covenantal relation with God—understood as the covenant of God with the "children of Noah." This covenant entails basic moral responsibilities that are incumbent on all human persons, such as prohibitions against murder and robbery. The extent to which these norms should be regarded as natural law, and in what sense of the term, has been debated vigorously.[9] Little attention has been given to ascertaining the precise application of the "Noahide" obligations. For Jews, the full scope of Jewish ethics, within the additional covenant of God with the Jewish people, is understood as both richer and more demanding than the minimalist requirements of Noahide ethics. For most of the past 2,000 years, few non-Jews have been interested in Jewish insights regarding their ethical responsibilities (see Introduction).

Views regarding the significance of universal human reason and experience vary widely across the three largest movements in the United States—Orthodox, Conservative, and Reform. All three of these movements have their roots in responses to modernity in nineteenth-century Germany. Representatives of each movement tend to see theirs as in many ways the most authentic Jewish approach, as well as the path offering the best prospects for the future. Each movement is complex and includes a broad range of stances, although some generalizations can provide a sense of tendencies within each.

Claims of universal reason and human experience tend to be strongest in Reform Judaism, the most left-wing of the largest movements in the United States. For classical Reform Judaism as it emerged in the nineteenth century, ethical truth was defined largely by liberal thought and progressive Western culture—in particular, Kant's ethics of reason. Where traditional Jewish ethics agreed with the ethics of reason, Jews could be proud of the pioneering contribution of their religion. In areas of disagreement, Judaism should change to better accord with ethical truth as defined by reason. The Reform commitment to reason and universal ethics has remained powerful but has become more nuanced in recent decades. Social and intellectual developments have called into question the easy identification of Western values with objective truth. The Holocaust in particular and broader social currents more generally have cast doubt on the inevitability of human progress and the obvious superiority of contemporary secular thought. Many Reform thinkers have come to understand their sense of identity and accompanying ethical responsibilities not only as generically human but also as shaped in part by community and covenantal responsibilities. This understanding has led to renewed attention to traditional Jewish teachings. Nevertheless, the commitment to human experience and universal reason remains powerful.[10]

Orthodox Judaism—the most right-wing of the three major movements—developed as a movement in response to Reform. Although modernity may bring benefits, in the Orthodox view the Enlightenment and modern thought pose threats to the integrity of Judaism. Orthodox Judaism emphasizes revelation and tradition as the decisive guides for Jewish ethics. J. David Bleich, for example, acknowledges that "basic moral values are universal and not contingent upon sectarian claims." Nevertheless, these values of reason are far less helpful than the norms of revelation in discerning ethical responsibility. "A person who seeks to find answers [to bioethical problems] within the Jewish tradition can deal with such questions in only one way. He must examine them through the prism of Halakhah, for it is in the corpus of Jewish law as elucidated and transmitted from generation to generation that God has made His will known to man."[11]

Other Orthodox thinkers defend important roles for general ethical values and for aggadah in providing a spiritual context for halakhic action and supporting supererogatory actions and admirable character traits, beyond those that could be specified by halakhah.[12] The use of reason also is clearly present in the development and evaluation of halakhic arguments, and ethical judgments are informed by human experience.[13] Halakhah and tradition remain primary and generally enjoy a lexical priority over other concerns. That which is specified by halakhah remains obligatory.[14] Reason is valued—but within the boundaries of religion (as defined by revelation and tradition) alone.

The Conservative movement also developed as a traditionalist response to Reform, though of a more centrist sort. Conservative writings on issues such as those arising in contemporary health care tend to operate from within a halakhic framework, as do Orthodox writings, but with greater attention to human experience and reason and to general ethical values. The primary source of ethical values in these works is the Jewish tradition—both in explicit statements of aggadah and in values implicit in halakhah (and aggadic narrative). Moreover, ethical reflections of non-Jewish thinkers—those of health care professionals, and of thinkers in general bioethics, philosophy, and varied religious traditions—are considered as well. Such sources are not regarded as determinative of Jewish ethics, and in some cases contrasts are drawn between Jewish and other views. Nevertheless, Conservative thinkers acknowledge, discuss, and learn from these sources.[15] Conservative writers devote attention to varied sources of guidance, including sacred texts, tradition, ethical values, theological concepts, contemporary circumstances, and the needs of individuals and the Jewish community. The best way to realize and balance these values is a complex, often disputed matter, even within the movement.[16]

Scripture and Tradition

In classical Jewish approaches, tradition and Scripture (as read by tradition) are central to ethics. Jewish thinkers exhibit a wide variety of views about the way in which the Bible—in particular, the Torah—represents God's word. Most Orthodox writers consider the text of the written Torah (Genesis through Deuteronomy) to have been presented by God to Moses, word by word and letter by letter, in a form identical to contemporary printed texts.[17] Reform thinkers tend to regard the Torah as divinely inspired in some sense, though largely the work of human hands. For Conservative writers, the Torah is divine in origin but is shaped significantly by human reception, transmission, and interpretation.[18]

As in Catholic thought, for Judaism Scripture and tradition represent distinct but complementary aspects of God's revelation. Central to tradition is oral Torah, which is classically understood both as the interpretation and development of the Biblical text and as a parallel divine communication, accompanying the written text, that was faithfully transmitted in oral form through many generations.[19]

Since late antiquity, numerous works of "oral Torah" have been given written form. Together these works constitute central resources for deliberation in bioethics and other areas. The *Mishnah* (meaning "study") was compiled early in the third century of the Common Era (c.e.) by Rabbi Judah Hanasi; it presented material that developed and was transmitted orally over the preceding centuries.[20] Another type of literature is represented by *midrash* ("search"): creative and interpretive commentaries on the Hebrew Bible.[21] In many ways the Talmud (like Mishnah, a term meaning "study") is the central work of the halakhic tradition. It records commentary on and discussion stemming from the Mishnah, developing over the centuries following compilation of the Mishnah. The Babylonian Talmud, which was compiled in Babylonia (present-day Iraq) in the sixth and seventh centuries c.e., often is referred to simply as "the Talmud."[22] Three types of post-Talmudic literature offer the most significant contributions to the fabric of Jewish law. One genre represents commentaries on the Talmud.[23] A second major genre is the *responsa*—in Hebrew *teshuvot* (singular: *teshuvah*, "response"). These *responsa* are the halakhic decisions of rabbinic authorities, addressing specific issues or cases; collectively they constitute the case law of Judaism. A third genre is represented by legal codes. Codes are not formally enacted but come to be recognized as authoritative—similar to the way in which the *Oxford English Dictionary* or *Encyclopaedia Britannica* have come to be recognized as authoritative. The first major systematic codification was produced by Moses Maimonides (Rabbi Moshe ben Maimon, also known as Rambam) in the twelfth century and is known as the *Mishneh Torah* ("repetition of the teaching"). The most authoritative code of law is the *Shulḥan Arukh* ("set table"), written by Rabbi Joseph Karo in the sixteenth century. Karo's code reflects Sephardic practices—those of Jews historically associated with Spain and the Mediterranean. Karo's text is published with interspersed glosses by Rabbi Moses Isserles, termed the *Mapah* ("tablecloth" for the set table), which reflect the customs of Ashkenazic Jews—those historically associated with Germany and Eastern Europe.[24]

Orthodox Judaism tends to present itself as continuing the unchanged Judaism of the past. Torah in general, and halakhah in particular, is essentially unchanging. As noted above, the text of the written Torah is regarded as identical to that presented by God to Moses. Oral Torah is understood primarily in terms of its articulation in the Talmud (based on material communicated by God to Moses) and received now as tradition from the past. Although new situations may call for thoughtful application of past precedents, Orthodox leaders tend to emphasize the need for caution and a desire to minimize change. Tendencies to emphasize the role of received tradition over reason, halakhah over aggadah, and stringency over flexibility are common in Orthodoxy. An essentially unchanging halakhah presents definitive requirements for Jewish ethics.

Conservative thinkers agree with their Orthodox colleagues that halakhah plays a definitive role in Jewish life and Jewish ethics. Yet halakhah has developed over time, through gradual evolution, and by means of textual and judicial interpretation. Such development, by such means, should continue; the model is one of "tradition and change."[25] Determination of which developments are appropriate is made primarily by rabbinic leadership, though there also is an appeal to a broader communal sense—analogous to the Roman Catholic *sensus fidei*.[26] Conservative writers characteristically attend to the historical development of halakhah. Although Torah is eternal, it develops in a way that manifests its strength and vitality as a living tradition. Past sources are read diachronically, tracing streams within the tradition and often finding divergent tendencies as well as ongoing development. Development has been, and should continue to be, organic, gradual, and evolutionary.[27]

Reform Judaism as it emerged in the nineteenth century understood the essential truths of Judaism to be unchanging: monotheism and a universalist ethic of love of neighbor. Other aspects of Judaism, including halakhah and traditional expressions of the oral Torah, are at best secondary and readily changeable. According to the Pittsburgh Platform of 1885:

> We hold that Judaism presents the highest conception of the God-idea as taught in our holy Scriptures and developed and spiritualized by the Jewish teachers in accordance with the moral and philo-

sophical progress of their respective ages. . . . We hold that all such Mosaic and Rabbinical laws as regulate diet, priestly purity and dress originated in ages and under the influence of ideas altogether foreign to our present mental and spiritual state. They fail to impress the modern Jew with a spirit of priestly holiness; their observance in our days is apt rather to obstruct than to further modern spiritual elevation.[28]

By the middle of the twentieth century Reform theologians had begun to accord greater significance to tradition, and in recent decades tradition has been identified as a valuable source of guidance. Nevertheless, it is clear that past teachings are not determinative of present responsibilities. "What keeps Judaism or any world view alive is its ability to grow and adapt," Eugene Borowitz writes. "For us, truth is, and always has been, something dynamic, a process of finding more adequate understanding."[29]

Authority

The issue of authority sharply divides the three major movements of Judaism. Classically, individuals seeking to follow Jewish ethics would be guided by a variety of influences, including narratives, rituals, exhortations to virtue, maxims, and communal customs. A central source of guidance would be halakhah. Traditional halakhah, like secular case law, uses analogies with precedent cases to decide new cases. Compared to other legal systems, halakhah is markedly open-ended, decentralized, and religiously sensitive; it is a legal system nonetheless.[30] The paramount authority in discerning halakhic guidance in a given case is the rabbi. Likewise, religious authority for the community as a whole is provided by rabbinic leadership. For most of the past two millennia, leadership has been decentralized, resting with various rabbis in local communities. Classically, positions were articulated by individual rabbis whose authority came to be recognized by their colleagues and their communities. Leaders of various academies, as well as rabbis of cities and communities, enjoyed significant authority; most generally deferred to tradition and current consensus. On the whole, then, the authority has been more closely akin to the Catholic magisterium of the Middle Ages than that of recent centuries. The authority of the rabbi in particular cases is somewhat analogous to the role of the priest in judging actions in the sacrament of penance.[31]

For most contemporary Orthodox thinkers, the traditional authority of the rabbi should be maintained. Advocating the centrality of rabbinic authority for particular bioethical decisions, Bleich asserts that patients and health care professionals alike lack the knowledge and objectivity required for sound decisions:

> The rabbinic tradition was fully cognizant of these factors . . . in its demand that the medical data be placed before a competent rabbinic authority prior to initiation of hazardous therapy or withholding of life-supporting measures. The rabbi serves as a legal arbiter and as an ethicist, a qualified expert capable of dispassionate examination of the data and of reaching a determination based upon the legal and ethical principles of his moral tradition.[32]

In sharp contrast, Reform writers emphasize the authority of each autonomous individual. Throughout the history of Reform Judaism, autonomy has been central to the articulation of Jewish ethics. Autonomy has taken various forms: a Kantian sense of the individual following dictates of universal reason; an individual liberty right of choice; a complex Jewish self, authentically making choices that reflect an identity that is significantly shaped by community and covenant with God.[33]

In recent decades, some Reform thinkers have accepted an increased role for halakhah in offering guidance to individuals, but individual autonomy remains predominant. Because of the unprecedented nature of many developments in health care ethics, traditional precedents may be too remote to offer extensive guidance. Even more basic is a commitment to the ultimate right of individuals to make autonomous decisions. An advocate of a "covenantal" approach argues that Jewish ethics should emphasize this right, rather than seeking to determine objective moral requirements.

> The rabbi could certainly occupy a legitimate role as consultant and could provide the patient, the family, and the physician with information drawn from the precedents of Jewish tradition on this matter. The patient, in the end, might well choose to follow them.

However, and this is the crucial point, it is the patient who would be empowered to make this decision. . . . The person's autonomy as a covenantal creature standing in relationship with God would ultimately be affirmed as the highest value in the system.[34]

Conservative writers generally seek a balance between the authority of the individual and that of his or her rabbi. In general, the authority of halakhah and the rabbinic decisor is primary. There are attempts, though, to emphasize and expand traditional warrants for individual choice. Avram Reisner relates the Talmudic account of Rabbi Judah Hanasi refusing the treatment prescribed by his physician, and refusing also the second proposed treatment, before accepting the physician's third suggestion. He concludes that "this realm of patient autonomy, then, does not reach quite as far as proposed by the secular ethicists. But it effectively controls most of the significant decisions to be made in treating the critically ill. . . . Save the decision to seek death, we function here almost exclusively within the realm of patient autonomy."[35]

Elliot Dorff criticizes the dominance of autonomy in Reform thought. This approach, he writes, threatens anarchy and the dissipation of community and "robs individuals of precisely what they seek when they turn to religion for guidance in these matters, for it tells them to seek God and decide for themselves." At the same time, Dorff accords a legitimate role to individual autonomy and, in fact, proclaims a right of conscientious dissent—although this right is to be exercised relatively infrequently. "Individuals retain the obligation to examine any law or ruling for its morality and to disobey all laws and rulings which are immoral on their face," Dorff writes. "Jewish law . . . asserts that God's law is just and good, and it bids us obey the rabbis' interpretation of that law in each generation; but it also requires that we go beyond the letter of the law and even disobey it when it—or a given interpretation of it—is mean-spirited or downright immoral."[36]

The balance of subjective and objective authority is a point of contention among Jewish writers. Almost all would agree, however, on the importance of the individual taking account of objective norms in formulating his or her own judgment. These norms are formulated on the basis of traditional texts, together with the reflections of reason.

Rules and General Values

A central issue in both Catholicism and Judaism is the relationship between general ethical values, such as human well-being, and specific moral norms. For some thinkers, general values are foundational and determine the shape of ethics. These values may be regarded as expressing love of neighbor. They typically fit as well with a general sense of consequentialism or with understandings of human dignity and respect for persons associated with Kant and his followers. On this view, specific moral prohibitions and requirements that fail to serve these general values may—in fact must—be modified. Such positions may be found among left-of-center Catholic moral theologians and among many thinkers in Reform Judaism.[37]

For others, decisive authority is accorded to the specific moral prohibitions and requirements articulated by the tradition or understood by the tradition to represent the demands of reason and natural law. These norms must be followed both because in some sense they represent objective moral truth or the will of God and because they represent the surest and perhaps the only way to achieve those general ethical values that all espouse. Moses Maimonides articulated such a view in his twelfth-century *Guide of the Perplexed*.[38] In more recent times, Pope Pius XII reflected a similar outlook in condemning artificial insemination. "We must never forget this: It is only the procreation of a new life according to the will and plan of the Creator which brings with it—to an astonishing degree of perfection—the realization of the desired ends. This is, at the same time, in harmony with the dignity of the marriage partners, with their body and spiritual nature, and with the normal and happy development of the child."[39] Violating established particular moral norms in pursuit of general values not only entails actions that are wrong in themselves but is self-defeating. Most Orthodox Jewish authorities would agree.

Finally, in each faith community there are some thinkers who seek to articulate a range of intermediate positions in which established norms have presumptive weight in ethical deliberation but in some cases may be reshaped, in light of basic values of the faith tradition and ongoing human reason and experience. Proponents present such views as appropriately combining "continuity and change."[40] These views may be found among moral theologians such as Richard

McCormick and Lisa Sowle Cahill, as well as among many thinkers within Judaism's Conservative movement.

Conclusion: Roman Catholic and Jewish Methodologies

Both Roman Catholicism and Judaism recognize several sources of guidance, including human experience and reason, Scripture, tradition, and respected teaching authority. For both traditions, these sources cannot fundamentally disagree because all ultimately reflect the same truth; accordingly, each source is properly understood in light of the others. In both traditions, the issue of authority has become a matter of sharp dispute (although in Judaism there is no centralized teaching authority akin to the Roman Catholic magisterium). Scripture, however defined, plays a similar role in moral analysis in both traditions. Scripture is read not as an independent document (or, at least, not only as such) but through the eyes of the present and historical community. In addition, Scripture functions primarily to provide fundamental values and to furnish effective quotations in driving home a position. Detailed analysis of Scripture generally receives less attention than tradition or reason in the formulation of specific ethical judgments.

In both Jewish and Roman Catholic ethics, reason and tradition work in tandem. In Judaism, however, tradition is central. Normative analysis of specific issues—of the sort most typical in contemporary bioethics—classically centers on halakhah, or Jewish law. A writer typically will cite earlier sources and draw analogies with precedents.[41] The model entails applying the tradition's guidance to the case at hand or, in unusual cases, showing how modification of accepted practice is appropriate, based on principles of the tradition itself. The use of reason is clearly present, and ethical judgments are informed by human experience.[42] These influences often are implicit, however. Tradition is privileged, and even claims that may seem to an outside observer to be motivated by reason and experience may be ascribed to tradition.

The converse is found in Roman Catholic moral theology. Normative analysis of specific issues generally centers on natural law. A writer is likely to make arguments based on human reason and experience, examining particular patterns found in creation, along with natural or ontic goods. The model entails applying the values of human nature, or the human person adequately considered, to the case at hand. The use of tradition is clearly present, informing readings of nature and the human person.[43] This influence often is implicit, however. Natural law is privileged, and even claims that may seem to an outside observer to be motivated by tradition (and the magisterium) may be ascribed to human reason and natural law.

The centrality of tradition and natural law, respectively, in Jewish and Catholic thought is reflected as well in the methodological disputes within each community. In Catholicism, natural law provides the dominating framework of discourse that is at once shared and contested by Catholic thinkers; the central disputes have tended to focus on natural law and its significance. According to critics, classical modes of Catholic thought are marked by physicalism, with excessive focus on the biological and physical. Nature has been improperly understood as static and immutable; there has been insufficient attention to the dynamics of historical development or to personal and spiritual values, including individual freedom and interpersonal relations. Some thinkers advocate personalism as a better approach in areas such as bioethics. Some theologians respond that although such spiritual concerns are important and may have received less than proper attention in the past, physical and biological aspects also are part of persons and nature and may not be violated. Spiritual and interpersonal values are to be pursued, but only within the confines set by consistency with physical and biological patterns of the natural law. Still other thinkers try to fashion mediating approaches, generating a methodological spectrum. In addition to disputes about what natural law should mean, there are disputes about how other sources of moral guidance should influence ethical decisions.[44]

Somewhat similarly, traditional texts—especially halakhic works— constitute the shared and contested terrain of Jewish ethics. According to critics, classical modes of Jewish thought are marked by legalism or formalism, with excessive focus on rules and precedents. Halakhah has been improperly understood as static and immutable; there has been insufficient attention to the dynamics of historical development or to personal and spiritual values, including individual freedom and interpersonal relations. A more dynamic and flexible approach, which some thinkers have termed "covenantal," is advocated as a better approach in areas such as bioethics. Some theologians respond that although such spiritual concerns are important and may have received less than proper attention in the past, the rules and precedents of halakhic authority also are central to Jewish ethics and the covenantal relationship with God, and these norms may not be violated. Spiritual and interpersonal values are to be pursued, but only within the confines set by consistency with requirements of traditional halakhic sources. Still other thinkers try to fashion mediating approaches, generating a methodological spectrum. In addition to disputes about what halakhah should mean, there are disputes about how other sources of moral guidance should influence ethical decisions.[45]

Roman Catholicism and Judaism are rich and complex traditions, extending back to ancient times and marked today by significant internal debates. I have attempted to provide a general survey and initial orientation to ethical reasoning in the two traditions. In the following chapters I attempt to fill in the sketch by examining deliberations regarding specific issues of bioethics.

Notes

1. Significant material from this section is adapted from my introduction to *Life and Death Responsibilities in Jewish Biomedical Ethics*, ed. Aaron L. Mackler (New York: Jewish Theological Seminary of America, Finkelstein Institute, 2000), 1–14.

2. According to one challenging but rich statement, "Even that which a student in the future would teach in the presence of his teacher was already said to Moses at Sinai" (Jerusalem Talmud, *Peah* 17a). See also Babylonian Talmud, *Menaḥot* 29b.

3. Ethical responsibilities in this section include positive obligations to revere parents, to leave corners of one's field unharvested for the poor to take, and to maintain honest weights for commerce and prohibitions against stealing and standing idly by as the blood of one's fellow is shed. These provisions are intermixed with injunctions that could be characterized as ritual: to observe the Sabbath, not to worship idols, not to eat meat from sacrifices on the wrong day (Leviticus 19).

4. Abraham Joshua Heschel, *God in Search of Man: A Philosophy of Judaism* (New York: Farrar, Straus and Giroux, 1955), 287.

5. See, for example, Louis E. Newman, "Ethics as Law, Law as Religion: Reflections on the Problem of Law and Ethics in Judaism," in *Contemporary Jewish Ethics and Morality*, ed. Elliot N. Dorff and Louis E. Newman (New York: Oxford University Press, 1995), 79–93, and Elliot Dorff, "A Methodology for Jewish Medical Ethics," 161–76 of the same volume. "Halakhah is God's gift to us, an expression of God's love. Similarly, our adherence to Halakhah is an act of love for God on our part. It is, in fact, the primary way in which God and the Jewish people exhibit their love for each other" (*Emet Ve-Emunah: Statement of Principles of Conservative Judaism* [New York: Jewish Theological Seminary of America, Rabbinical Assembly, United Synagogue of America, 1988], 22).

6. Naḥmanides, commentary to Lev. 19:2, in *Perushei haTorah l'Rabenu Moshe ben Naḥman*, ed. Chaim Dov Chavel, vol. 2 (Jerusalem: Mosad haRav Kook, 1960), 115.

7. In dealing with *tzedakah* (support for the poor), for example, halakhah prescribes fixed amounts that individuals are obligated to give, whereas aggadah emphasizes the importance of generosity and compassion.

8. Heschel, *God in Search of Man,* 341.

9. See David Novak, *Natural Law in Judaism* (Cambridge: Cambridge University Press, 1998); Louis E. Newman, *Past Imperatives: Studies in the History and Theory of Jewish Ethics* (Albany: State University of New York Press, 1999), 117–38.

10. See Eugene B. Borowitz, *Exploring Jewish Ethics* (Detroit: Wayne State University Press, 1990), esp. 22–23, 26–36, 176–92. On the relation of Jewish ethics to universal reason, see David Novak, "Bioethics and the Contemporary Jewish Community," *Hastings Center Report* 20, no. 3 (1990 suppl.): 14–17; Newman, *Past Imperatives*, 101–15, 205–20; Noam Zohar, *Alternatives in Jewish Bioethics* (Albany: State University of New York Press, 1997), 1–16; Laurie Zoloth-Dorfman, "Face to Face, Not Eye to Eye: Further Conversations on Jewish Medical Ethics," *Journal of Clinical Ethics* 6 (1995): 222–31.

11. J. David Bleich, "The *A Priori* Component of Bioethics," in *Jewish Bioethics*, ed. Fred Rosner and J. David Bleich (New York: Sanhedrin, 1979), xix.

12. See Aharon Lichtenstein, "Does Jewish Tradition Recognize an Ethic Independent of Halakha?" in *Contemporary Jewish Ethics*, ed. Menachem Marc Kellner (New York: Sanhedrin, 1978), 102–23.

13. See Zohar, *Alternatives in Jewish Bioethics*, 8–10.

14. See Lichtenstein, "Ethic Independent of Halakha?"

15. See Mackler, *Life and Death Responsibilities*, 8.

16. See, for example, Seymour Siegel, ed., *Conservative Judaism and Jewish Law* (New York: Rabbinical Assembly, 1977); Dorff, "Methodology for Jewish Medical Ethics"; Joel Roth, *The Halakhic Process: A Systemic Analysis* (New York: Jewish Theological Seminary of America, 1986); Gordon Tucker, "God, the Good, and Halakhah," *Judaism* 38 (1989): 365–76; Aaron L. Mackler, "Cases and Principles in Jewish Bioethics: Toward a Holistic Model," in Dorff and Newman, *Contemporary Jewish Ethics and Morality*, 177–93.

17. See Norman Lamm's statement in *The Condition of Jewish Belief* (New York: Macmillan, 1966), 124–25.

18. See Neil Gillman, *Sacred Fragments: Recovering Theology for the Modern Jew* (Philadelphia: Jewish Publication Society, 1990).

19. The classical proclamation regarding the transmission of oral Torah is found in the Mishnah, *Avot* 1:1 (third century C.E.). Later views of halakhic exegesis as primarily development or received tradition are discussed in Jay M. Harris, *How Do We Know This? Midrash and the Fragmentation of Modern Judaism* (Albany: State University of New York Press, 1995). On parallels in Catholic thought, see the discussion above in chapter 2 and *Dei Verbum*, nn. 8–12, in *Vatican Council II: The Conciliar and Post Conciliar Documents*, new revised ed., ed. Austin Flannery (Northport, N.Y.: Costello, 1996), 754–57. An analogous view to classical understandings of oral Torah as received tradition, parallel to Scripture, is found in the "Decree Concerning the Canonical Scriptures" of the Council of Trent (sixteenth century). According to the Council, the Gospel was promulgated personally by Jesus Christ, "as the source at once of all saving truth and rules of conduct. . . . These truths and rules are contained [both] in the written books and in the unwritten traditions, which, received by the Apostles from the mouth of Christ Himself . . . have come down to us, transmitted as it were from hand to hand" (*Canons and Decrees of the Council of Trent*, trans. H. J. Schroeder [St. Louis: B. Herder, 1941], 17).

20. On the classical texts of oral Torah, see Mackler, *Life and Death Responsibilities*, 10–12; David M. Feldman, *Birth Control in Jewish Law*, rev. ed. (Northvale, N.J.: Jason Aronson, 1998), 3–18. The Mishnah consists primarily of a listing of halakhic positions attributed to different halakhic authorities—especially those of the second century C.E.—organized topically in several *masekhtot* (singular: *masekhet*, tractate). The *Tosefta* ("addition") is a supplemental and less authoritative collection of materials from this period, edited in the fourth or fifth century C.E.

21. Prominent collections of halakhic midrash are the *Mekhilta* (on Exodus), *Sifra* (on Leviticus), and *Sifre* (on Numbers and Deuteronomy); these *midrashim* were compiled in the fourth or fifth century C.E., though

they contain earlier material. Numerous works of aggadic midrash developed over subsequent centuries.

22. The Jerusalem Talmud, also referred to as the "Talmud of the Land of Israel" or "Palestinian Talmud," is a less authoritative work that was compiled in northern Israel in the fifth century C.E.

23. The best-known and most influential commentary is that of Rashi (Rabbi Shlomo Yitzhaki, eleventh century C.E.). This commentary is printed together with the Talmudic text in standard editions of the Talmud. Also appearing in the standard edition are commentaries of Rashi's grandchildren and others known as the *Tosafot* ("additions"). Numerous additional commentaries have been developed over the centuries as well.

24. An additional influential work was the *Arba'ah Turim* ("four columns") of Rabbi Jacob ben Asher. Karo's *Shulḥan Arukh* draws on his monumental commentary (the *Beit Yosef*) on this work.

25. See Mordecai Waxman, ed., *Tradition and Change: The Development of Conservative Judaism* (New York: Rabbinical Assembly, 1958); Elliot N. Dorff, *Conservative Judaism: Our Ancestors to Our Descendants*, rev. ed. (New York: United Synagogue of Conservative Judaism, 1996).

26. "Since then the interpretation of Scripture or the Secondary Meaning [oral Torah] is mainly a product of changing historical influences, it follows that the centre of authority is actually removed from the Bible and placed in some *living body*, which, by reason of its being in touch with the ideal aspirations and the religious needs of the age, is best able to determine the nature of the Secondary Meaning. This living body, however, is not represented by any section of the nation, or any corporate priesthood, or Rabbihood, but by the collective conscience of Catholic Israel as embodied in the Universal Synagogue. . . . This Synagogue, the only true witness to the past, and forming in all ages the sublimest expression of Israel's religious life, must also retain its authority as the sole true guide for the present and the future" (Solomon Schechter, "Introduction to Studies in Judaism: First Series," in *Studies in Judaism: A Selection* [Philadelphia: Jewish Publication Society, 1958], 15–16; emphasis in original).

27. See, e.g., Dorff, "A Methodology for Jewish Medical Ethics," 164. Conservative writers would tend to characterize tradition in a manner akin to Richard McCormick (see chapter 1). Like McCormick, they would characterize themselves as representing the "extreme middle" (Richard McCormick, *Health and Medicine in the Catholic Tradition* [New York: Crossroad, 1987], 3).

28. "The Pittsburgh Platform," in *The Jew in the Modern World*, ed. Paul M. Mendes-Flohr and Jehuda Reinharz (New York: Oxford University Press, 1980), 371–72.

29. Eugene B. Borowitz, *Liberal Judaism* (New York: Union of American Hebrew Congregations, 1984), 13–14. "The Jewish self, through Covenant, is historically rooted. . . . Much of what Jews once did is likely to commend itself to us as what we ought to do. More, since their sense of the Covenant was comparatively fresh, strong and steadfast, while ours is often uncertain, weak and faltering, we will substantially rely on their guidance in determining our Jewish duty. But not to the point of dependency or passivity of will. Not only is our situation in many respects radically different from theirs but our identification of maturity with the proper exercise of agency (in Covenantal context for a Jew) requires us on occasion to dissent from what our tradition has taught or enjoined" (Borowitz, *Exploring Jewish Ethics*, 183).

30. See Newman, *Past Imperatives*, 103–5.

31. As noted by James M. Gustafson, "It is not unreasonable to suggest that this role of priest is more similar historically to one aspect of the office of the rabbi in traditional Judaism than it is to the role of the Protestant minister. Both the priest and the rabbi function as teachers of morality. They are the instructors of their congregations in the requirements of morality and, indeed, of moral law. The rabbi . . . has functioned as a judge in disputed claims made in accordance with the halakhah. To be a wise judge he must know the law, just as the priest must know the moral and canon law to be a sound and wise confessor. To make judgments, both the priest and the rabbi exercise their capacities to reason—granted, in quite different ways. For both, however, a body of law (or quasi-legal moral theology) is necessary if they are to function in their professional roles" (*Protestant and Roman Catholic Ethics: Prospects for Rapprochement* [Chicago: University of Chicago Press, 1978], 2).

32. J. David Bleich, "The Obligation to Heal in the Judaic Tradition," *Jewish Bioethics*, ed. Fred Rosner and J. David Bleich (New York: Sanhedrin, 1979), 37. Similarly, after noting the possibility of forgoing life-sustaining treatment in some circumstances, Immanuel Jakobovits stipulates, "This assumes that every single such case would be submitted to competent medical judgment in consultation with equally competent moral authorities—rabbis in the case of those who submit to Jewish law—and that each case is individually judged to comply with these careful definitions as given" ("Ethical Problems Regarding the Termination of Life," in *Jewish Values in Bioethics*, ed. Levi Meier [New York: Human Sciences Press, 1986], 91). See also David H. Ellenson, "How to Draw Guidance from a Heritage: Jewish Approaches to Mortal Choices" in Dorff and Newman, *Contemporary Jewish Ethics and Morality*, 135.

33. See Borowitz, *Exploring Jewish Ethics*, 176–92.

34. Ellenson, "How to Draw Guidance from a Heritage," 138.

35. Avram I. Reisner, "Care for the Terminally Ill: Halakhic Concepts and Values," in Mackler, *Life and Death Responsibilities in Jewish Biomedical Ethics*, 250–51, citing *Bava Metzia* 85b.

36. Elliot Dorff, "End Stage Medical Care: Halakhic Concepts and Values," in Mackler, *Life and Death Responsibilities in Jewish Biomedical Ethics*, 310–11; idem, "A Methodology for Jewish Medical Ethics," in Dorff and Newman, *Contemporary Jewish Ethics and Morality*, 164–65.

37. E.g., Margaret A. Farley, "An Ethic for Same-Sex Relations," in *Readings in Moral Theology, no. 8: Dialogue about Catholic Sexual Teaching*, ed. Charles E. Curran and Richard McCormick (Mahwah, N.J.: Paulist, 1993), 338–46.

38. Moses Maimonides, *The Guide of the Perplexed*, pt. III, ch. 26–27, trans. Shlomo Pines (Chicago: University of Chicago Press, 1963), 506–12.

39. Pope Pius XII, "Address to the Fourth International Convention of Catholic Physicians" (September 1949), in Farley, *Readings in Moral Theology, no. 8*, 224. Likewise, William E. May asserts a general principle that each human person should be valued, or "wanted," and continues, "The only way to shape human choices and human actions—and through them human persons and human societies—so that human beings will be wanted as they ought to be wanted is by ordering them in accordance with true and objective norms" ("The Liberating Truth of Catholic Teaching on Sexual Morality," in Farley, *Readings in Moral Theology, no. 8*, 513). See similarly Benedict M. Ashley and Kevin D. O'Rourke, *Health Care Ethics: A Theological Analysis*, 4th ed. (Washington, D.C.: Georgetown University Press, 1997), 246. Bernard Häring articulates the general importance of moral norms in terms that many Jewish thinkers would find familiar: "Commandment and law are and always must be central ideas in the Christian moral teaching. . . . The commandments of God are words of the divine Love addressed to us, expressed in the great command of love. And true fulfillment of the command is the obedient response of love, obedient love" (*The Law of Christ*, vol. 1, trans. Edwin G. Kaiser [Westminster, Md.: Newman, 1963], 42).

40. Richard McCormick, "Therapy or Tampering? The Ethics of Reproductive Technology," *America* 153 (1985): 400. The phrase "tradition and change" is a motto of the Conservative movement of Judaism (e.g., Waxman, *Tradition and Change*).

41. Similar case-based patterns of reasoning appear in Roman Catholic ethics, where they are associated with casuistry. See Albert R. Jonsen and Stephen Toulmin, *The Abuse of Casuistry: A History of Moral Reasoning* (Berkeley: University of California Press, 1988); James F. Keenan and Thomas

A. Shannon, eds., *The Context of Casuistry* (Washington, D.C.: Georgetown University Press, 1995).

42. The balance between reason and tradition varies among Jewish ethical writers, and the use of reason tends to become more explicit and often more powerful as one moves toward the left on the methodological spectrum. Reason plays a significant though secondary role even in classical traditional writings. See discussion above and Zohar, 8–10.

43 As noted by Lisa Sowle Cahill, "Even contemporary natural law thinkers are increasingly ready to recognize the 'postmodern' emphasis on contextualism, particularity, and tradition, and hence to recognize that Catholic natural law thinking, while aiming at the 'universal,' is worked out within a historically particular religious tradition: Christianity as Catholicism" ("Can Theology Have a Role in 'Public' Bioethical Discourse?" *Hastings Center Report* 20, no. 4 [1990, suppl.]: 13).

44. E.g., David F. Kelly, *The Emergence of Roman Catholic Medical Ethics in North America* (New York: Edward Mellen Press, 1979); idem, *Critical Care Ethics: Treatment Decisions in American Hospitals* (Kansas City: Sheed and Ward, 1991); Ashley and O'Rourke, *Health Care Ethics*, esp. 156–76.

45. Ellenson, "How to Draw Guidance from a Heritage"; Lichtenstein, "Ethic Independent of Halakha?" 114–17; Mackler, "Cases and Principles in Jewish Bioethics" and additional essays in Dorff and Newman, *Contemporary Jewish Ethics and Morality*, 129–76.

Chapter 3

Euthanasia and Assisted Suicide

IN THIS CHAPTER I EXAMINE JEWISH AND CATHOLIC approaches to the issues of active euthanasia and assisted suicide. I survey writings on the topic, moving generally from right to left—beginning with arguments against, then considering arguments for, euthanasia.

To an extent that is remarkable in light of methodological differences at the theoretical level, theologians in the two traditions frame the issues in similar ways and identify similar sets of specific concerns; although such similarities are evident throughout this volume, they are particularly striking with regard to this topic. A spectrum of responses on euthanasia and assisted suicide emerges in each tradition. Substantively, the range of Jewish positions tends to overlap with and extend somewhat to the right of Catholic views, although this rightward leaning is less prominent here than on the related issue of forgoing life-sustaining treatment (see chapter 4).

Writers in the two traditions offer similar reasons for their views. Jewish and Catholic theologians share many basic values and generally express similar understandings of God, humanity, and the world—often citing the same Scriptural texts. There is some tendency for Catholic thinkers to place greater emphasis on natural law and teleological concerns, including a normative model of a spiritually good death. Appeals to tradition and examination of textual sources tend to be more prominent among Jewish writers. These tendencies reflect general characteristics of the religions, as noted in chapters 1 and 2. Jewish ethics has long focused on tradition and halakhah, though reason and experience have always been part of the process as well; Catholic ethics has focused on reason and natural law teleology, though tradition has been recognized as an important source of authority (see chapters 1 and 2). I consider some possible explanations for the convergence of the two traditions, as well as factors that may contribute to the differences between them. I also address briefly the significance of convergence and divergence between these traditions for practical ethics as practiced by moral thinkers within each faith community and generally in the context of contemporary societies such as the United States.

Opposition to Euthanasia

Most Catholic and Jewish writers oppose active euthanasia and assisted suicide. Opposition may be most vociferous toward the right of each spectrum, from magisterial documents and their consistent supporters in Catholic thought and from Orthodox rabbinic decisors in Judaism. Nevertheless, even thinkers who are more liberal on some issues, including proportionalists among Catholics and Conservative (centrist) and Reform (liberal) Jewish authorities—with some exceptions—tend to oppose euthanasia. For some thinkers, the most fundamental reason for opposing euthanasia is that it violates divine and human law. These writers cite biblical proclamations of God's prohibition of killing from Genesis 9 and Exodus 20. These prohibitions have been maintained by each tradition and have been applied consistently by the tradition to suicide and to the killing of persons who are suffering. Jewish and Catholic thinkers alike—especially those toward the right of the spectrum within each tradition—turn to traditional discussion of suicide for precedents for assisted suicide and euthanasia. Thomas Aquinas's classic statement provides a reference point for many Catholic thinkers: Suicide is wrong because it violates one's duties to oneself, to the community, and to God.[1] Similarly, Jewish thinkers appeal to prohibitions of suicide in classical legal codes such as the *Mishneh Torah* of Moses Maimonides and Joseph Karo's *Shulḥan Arukh*; suicide is included in the category of murder. Writers in each tradition argue that in some ways suicide is an especially grievous sin because it eliminates the possibility of future repentance.[2] Classical sources specify posthumous punishments for persons who commit suicide, including restrictions on their burial. Especially in recent times, such penalties seldom have been applied in practice.

There is a strong presumption that the individual committing suicide was not in full control of his or her actions—so guilt is mitigated subjectively, even though the deed is objectively wrong.[3]

An important reason for the prohibition against all killing, including suicide and euthanasia, is that these actions repudiate divine sovereignty. The basic prohibition—and this rationale—are central to the arguments of thinkers toward the right of the spectrum in each tradition. Killing oneself or others violates God's plan, which humans ought to respect. Our lives ultimately belong not to us but to God. As expressed in the U.S. Conference of Catholic Bishops' "Ethical and Religious Directives for Catholic Health Care Services," "We are not the owners of our lives and hence do not have absolute power over life. We have a duty to preserve our life and to use it for the glory of God."[4] In Thomas Aquinas's image, "a person who takes his own life sins against God, just as he who kills another's slave injures the slave's master." Similarly, traditional Jewish law prohibits individuals from injuring themselves or killing themselves, as well as injuring or killing others—even with the victim's consent. As explained by Eliezer Yehudah Waldenberg, "the life of man is not his possession, but the possession of the Holy One, Blessed be He." When there is conflict between the words of the master (God) and the disciple (man), one follows the words of the master.[5]

Acceptance of the traditional prohibition of suicide and euthanasia and grounding for this prohibition in divine sovereignty are found in some more centrist thinkers as well (though for centrists other considerations tend to be relatively more important). John Paris cites with approval the statement in the Vatican "Declaration on Euthanasia" that no one may ask to be killed or kill another because "only the Creator of life has the right to take away the life of the innocent."[6] Conservative rabbi Elliot Dorff expresses a similar view: "According to Judaism, God created and therefore owns the entire universe, including each person's body, and each of us therefore has a fiduciary responsibility to God to preserve our life and health."[7]

God's creation of humanity grounds not only God's dominion over human life but also the sacred and inviolable quality of that life. The narrative of Genesis 1 teaches that God created humans in God's image, endowing human life with basic and great value. For the Vatican Declaration, "Most people regard life as something sacred and hold that no one may dispose of it at will, but believers see in life something greater, namely a gift of God's love, which they are called upon to preserve and make fruitful."[8] Similarly, Orthodox rabbi Immanuel Jakobovits speaks of "the inviolable sanctity of human life."[9] Accordingly, two related arguments are offered against the claim that killing a patient may provide a benefit in some cases. First, killing a patient for his or her benefit would violate God's authority; second, it really would not provide a benefit to the patient. Aquinas argues:

> [1] the passage from this life to a more blessed one is, however, not a matter subject to man's free will, but to God's power. A man may not, therefore, kill himself in order to pass into the more blessed life. Similarly, [2] a man may not kill himself in order to escape from any of the miseries of this life. For, as Aristotle points out, the very worst and most fearful evil of this life is death. So to inflict death on oneself in order to escape from the miseries of this life is to take on a greater evil in order to avoid a lesser.[10]

Orthodox rabbi J. David Bleich presents a similarly two-pronged argument: [1] "Mercy-killing is proscribed as an unwarranted intervention in an area which must be governed only by God Himself"; furthermore, [2] "life accompanied by pain is . . . viewed as preferable to death."[11]

Jewish and Catholic writers emphasize the value of each human person, regardless of disabilities that may prevent human observers from appreciating this divinely recognized worth. For example, Catholics Jean deBlois and Kevin O'Rourke write, "The most telling argument against PAS [physician-assisted suicide] is based on the nature of our relationship to God. Human beings simply do not have dominion over the lives of innocent people. Human beings are not morally competent to decide that killing a person is the best way to alleviate his or her suffering, that he or she would be 'better off dead.'"[12] Dorff argues similarly: "The Jewish tradition . . . calls upon us to evaluate life from God's perspective. That means that the value of life does not depend on the level of one's abilities; it derives from the image of God embedded in us. The tradition thus strongly affirms the divine quality of the life of disabled people."[13]

For writers in each tradition there is a link between the central concerns of violation of divine authority and abuse of human persons.

As Pope John Paul II argues in *Evangelium Vitae*: "God alone has the power of life and death. . . . But he only exercises this power in accordance with a plan of wisdom and love. When man usurps this power, being enslaved by a foolish and selfish way of thinking, he inevitably uses it for injustice and death."[14] Remarkably similar concerns are expressed in a document from the Responsa Committee of the Central Conference of American Rabbis—the Reform (and most liberal) branch of Judaism: "It is an awesome and awful responsibility we take upon ourselves when we determine to kill a human being, even when our intentions are good and merciful. Such an action is the ultimate arrogance, for it declares that we are masters over the one thing—life itself—that our faith has always taught must be protected against our all-too-human tendency to manipulate, to mutilate, and to destroy."[15]

Catholic and Jewish writers note particular problems in contemporary societies, such as the United States, in distorting appreciation of human worth. *Evangelium Vitae* warns of "a cultural context frequently closed to the transcendent" and, indeed, a

> "culture of death," which is advancing above all in prosperous societies, marked by an attitude of excessive preoccupation with efficiency and which sees the growing number of elderly and disabled people as intolerable and too burdensome. These people are very often isolated by their families and by society, which are organized almost exclusively on the basis of productive efficiency, according to which a hopelessly impaired life no longer has any value.[16]

Likewise, Catholic Bernard Häring writes of the need to "override a utilitarian philosophy and strengthen the respect for each person."[17] Dorff similarly criticizes an ideology in the United States that "would have us think of ourselves in utilitarian terms, where our worth is a function of what we can do for ourselves and others."[18]

Another societal concern, expressed by thinkers toward the middle as well as the right of each spectrum, is excessive emphasis on autonomy (in the sense of individual free choice). Catholic Richard McCormick criticizes a cultural "absolutization of autonomy," with two "noxious offshoots":

> First, very little thought is then given to the values that ought to inform and guide the use of autonomy. Given such a vacuum, the

sheer fact that a choice is the patient's tends to be viewed as the sole right-making characteristic of the choice. Autonomy has become overstated and distorted. That overstatement translates into a total accommodation to the patient's values and wishes. If physician-assisted suicide is one of those wishes, well. . . . The second concomitant of absolutizing autonomy is an intolerance of dependence on others.[19]

Dorff similarly contrasts an American emphasis on liberty with the responsibility that Judaism teaches to live under God's authority.[20]

Opponents of euthanasia in each tradition argue that the apparent compassion of mercy killing is false and that there are better and more compassionate ways to respond to the suffering of severely ill and dying patients. According to *Evangelium Vitae*, "euthanasia must be called a *false mercy*, and indeed a disturbing 'perversion' of mercy. True 'compassion' leads to sharing another's pain; it does not kill the person whose suffering we cannot bear." Similarly, McCormick argues that "assisted suicide is a flight from compassion, not an expression of it. It should be suspect not because it is too hard, but because it is too easy."[21] A call for proper compassion, expressed in strikingly similar terms, likewise is found among Jewish writers such as Dorff: "In attending to the sick, we must assure that their physical needs are met and that their ending time in life is as psychologically, emotionally, and religiously meaningful as possible. Our compassion, in other words, must be expressed in these demanding ways rather than in acquiescing to a request for assistance in dying."[22]

Concretely, opponents of euthanasia (as well as proponents) argue for the importance of better pain relief. McCormick characterizes inadequate control of pain as a central factor that leads some people to support assisted suicide; he advocates better education and pain control. Similarly, the importance of supportive care and pain relief—palliative care—is emphasized by the bishops in the "Ethical and Religious Directives" and by Jewish writers such as Dorff. These writers generally endorse hospice and supportive care.[23]

Some writers argue that although suffering should be alleviated, it would be unrealistic to try to eliminate all suffering from human life and that suffering may even lead to valuable contributions in the grand scheme of things. According to the Vatican Declaration, "suffering, especially suffering during the last moments of life, has a special place in God's saving plan: It is in fact a sharing in Christ's passion and a union with the redeeming sacrifice which he offered in obedience to the Father's will."[24] McCormick endorses a more general appreciation of the value in suffering found in an Anglican document.

> The value of human life does not consist simply of a scale of plea- sure and pain. . . . The value of human life consists in a variety of virtues and graces as well as in pleasure. These together constitute man's full humanity. They grow in soil in which action and passion, doing and suffering, pleasure and pain are intermixed. What a man is consists not only of what he does, but also of how he endures. A fully human life is inevitably vulnerable, as every lover knows, and even suffering may by grace be woven into the texture of a larger humanity.[25]

Like McCormick, the Reform Jewish responsum expresses appre- ciation of the presence of suffering in human life:

> Pain and suffering are part and parcel of the human condition. . . . Even in debilitating illness, when our freedom of action is severely limited, we yet sanctify the divine name by *living* our relationship with God, by striving toward nobility of conduct and of purpose, by confronting our suffering with courage. To say this is not to ignore the agony of the dying but to recognize a fundamental truth: that even when we are dying we have the power to choose how we shall live. We can kill ourselves, thereby accepting the counsel of despair, or we can choose life, declaring through our actions that despite everything life—all of it—is blessed with the promise of ultimate meaning and fulfillment.[26]

Many opponents of euthanasia emphasize the legitimacy of for- going life-sustaining treatment in appropriate cases. Some thinkers toward the right of the Jewish spectrum express great caution and may even condemn most cases of forgoing treatment as similar to active euthanasia; in their view, such actions fail to appreciate the value of life or to fulfill the human obligation to save and prolong life.[27] Oth- ers note the potential legitimacy of forgoing treatment in some cases.[28] Centrist Jewish sources more clearly endorse the forgoing of treatment in appropriate cases and even criticize overtreatment. As Dorff writes, "far too many people with irreversible, terminal illnesses are subjected to futile, aggressive treatment," and "far too many people are finding that their express desire for life support to be withheld or withdrawn . . . is being ignored."[29] Catholic sources across a broad spectrum consistently support forgoing of disproportionate treatment and condemn the imposition of excessive treatment.[30] Indeed, many Catholic thinkers draw parallels between euthanasia on one hand and overtreatment on the other. Paris argues that a medical system that refuses to accept death and unduly prolongs dying leads to a desire for a technological "quick fix" when cure is not forthcoming.[31] Similarly, James Bresnahan advocates a balanced and "sober realism," navigating between the extremes of vitalism and active euthanasia.[32] The greater emphasis among Catholics than among Jews on condemning overtreatment correlates with the generally more conservative stance of Jewish thinkers on forgoing treatment (see chapter 4).

Thinkers in each tradition express concern that any societal acceptance of assisted suicide or euthanasia risks expansion to other cases, both by eroding the commitment of health care professionals to patients and more generally by diminishing support for weak and vulnerable persons in continuing to remain alive. For thinkers toward the right of each spectrum, these policy concerns often seem to be secondary and supportive of the central arguments that assisted suicide and euthanasia are intrinsically wrong. For those toward the center, policy considerations often appear predominant; absent these concerns, there might be more room for flexibility in interpreting the restrictions imposed by divine sovereignty, for example. Häring expresses concern with the effect of institutionalizing euthanasia on the relationship of physicians to patients. He also warns of the risk of dangerous developments of the sort associated with "slippery slope" arguments. Disabled and vulnerable persons "might be influenced by worry about the trouble they are causing their family." "Is a sense of guilt at being alive to be added to a feeling of resignation . . . at dying?"[33]

Such policy concerns are even more prominent among Jewish writers. Dorff warns that if assisted suicide is legalized,

> *permission* to take one's own life and to enlist the aid of others in doing so will quickly become all but an *obligation* to end the lives of those who have no reasonable hope for cure. Physicians, in the worst scenario, will be pressured by hospitals or health insurance compa-

nies to convince their patients that suicide is the best option. . . . The role of the physician as the patient's advocate thus becomes severely compromised. The same considerations apply to the patient's family members. If assisted suicide becomes a guaranteed constitutional right in U.S. law, patients will feel all the more pressed by their families to end their lives. . . . Legitimating assisted suicide thus dangerously shifts the burden of proof: Currently those who want to take a life must justify that course of action, but if assisted suicide becomes legal, those who refuse it will need to show why.[34]

Similarly, the Reform responsum argues that once active ending of life is accepted in some cases, it would be hard to deny this option in others. "So long as a person concludes that 'I do not want to live like this,' we would have no right to oppose that decision." The experience of the Netherlands suggests that nonobservance of rules limiting euthanasia is likely. "Indeed, the move from voluntary to involuntary euthanasia is a natural one; for once we have convinced ourselves that the absence of an identifiable standard of quality of life justifies the destruction of that life, why should we hold ourselves back from acting on that belief?"[35]

Catholic writers are much more likely than Jewish thinkers to oppose euthanasia as inconsistent with a model of a good death. Writers such as Bresnahan and McCormick present a normative approach to dying as fundamental to consideration of euthanasia. According to McCormick, "until our culture has a healthy Christian attitude toward death, it cannot trust the answers it gives and must give to the many extremely difficult questions involved in any acceptance of positive euthanasia."[36] More generally, Bresnahan claims that "nothing is more central to Catholic belief and practice than seeking, by anticipation, to deal well with one's own dying and with the dying of one's neighbor." Although Häring notes policy considerations opposing euthanasia, his central concern is that active choice of death would tend to "diminish the fullness of the free acceptance of death" and would be inconsistent with "the most truthful admission of our creaturely human existence."[37]

On the whole, Jewish writers exhibit a somewhat greater tendency to cite (religious) legal precedent and other texts from the tradition. Catholic writers exhibit a greater tendency to write in terms of teleology and the normative model of a good death. Nonetheless, opponents of euthanasia in both traditions utilize both reason and tradition, with some appeal to texts and central values emerging from Scripture. To an impressive extent, theologians in the two traditions frame the issues in similar ways and identify similar sets of specific concerns.

Arguments for Euthanasia

Some (generally liberal) members in each faith community accept euthanasia. This acceptance tends to be expressed with caution—as relatively rare exceptions to general rules against active killing, with a professed need for safeguards and careful development of public policy. Support for euthanasia generally is found only in academic theological writings, not in documents providing normative guidance for communities. For Catholicism, with its centralized magisterial authority, this observation almost goes without saying. Within Judaism, it is noteworthy that halakhic decisions approved by central bodies of the Conservative and Reform movements have opposed active euthanasia. Writings that support or at least offer reasons to allow euthanasia may be found among individual academics whose personal commitments are Reform, Conservative, and Orthodox.

Thinkers who present arguments for the acceptability of euthanasia ground these positions in the observation that although biological life generally is valuable, it is not the highest human value. As Catholic theologian Margaret Farley notes, "Human life has profound value; it is even holy. Yet death may sometimes be welcomed—if it is welcomed in a way that does not ignore or violate the requirement to respect and to value each person. . . . There are and will be rare circumstances, exceptional cases . . . in which the active taking of life may be justified."[38] Similarly, Reform rabbi Peter Knobel states:

> Judaism values the pursuit of health and the preservation of life as very important *mitzvot* [commandments]. . . . However, it is also clear in Judaism that biological life, while an important value, is not a supreme value which overrides all other considerations. Therefore, in extreme situations, the termination of human life is not considered a sin, but is in fact praiseworthy. The determining factor is whether the termination of life is consistent with the person as a being created *b'tzelem elohim* [in God's image].[39]

Each religious tradition has recognized circumstances in which one justifiably may choose to end life. Each tradition generally accepts the killing of an aggressor to protect innocent life, establishing the possibility of justifiable homicide.[40] Of special interest is traditional acceptance of (and praise for) martyrdom, which involves the death of an innocent person. For some supporters of euthanasia, the martyrdom paradigm is not helpful because the martyr is sacrificing his or her interests in the service of divine sovereignty.[41] Others, however, read the martyr paradigm more broadly. Conservative rabbi Byron Sherwin suggests that martyrdom offers

> precedents for taking one's own life and allowing oneself to be killed rather than to endure the physical torture that was frequently a martyr's fate. . . . What proves intriguing is the pertinence and the applicability that instances in which martyrs chose death to physical suffering, chose to accelerate their own death rather than to withstand physical agony, may have to the problem of euthanasia.[42]

Others read the example of martyrs as supporting a person's choosing death when he or she finds this choice necessary for his or her own sense of integrity. Thus, Farley argues that the obligation to preserve life may be limited by "personal integrity and moral or religious witness: For the martyr, life is less valuable than the integrity of her or his faith or moral commitments; it may also be of less value than witnessing to what is believed to be right or true." Knobel extends the paradigm a step further. Jewish acceptance of martyrdom shows that suicide "is permitted when continuing to live violates a fundamental principle of what life is all about." Martyrs "preferred death to a life which required them to live in a way that was inconsistent with their life plan."[43]

An important argument in favor of the possibility of euthanasia suggests that God's sovereignty does not necessarily forbid all acts of active killing. This line of argument is especially clear for a patient who is already dying. According to Catholic theologian Charles Curran, "precisely because the dying process has now begun, man's positive intervention is not an arrogant usurping of the role of God but rather in keeping with the process of dying which is now encompassing the person." More generally, the acceptability of forgoing life-sustaining treatment suggests that "man does have some dominion over the dying process."[44] Similarly, Jewish academic Noam Zohar argues that accepting God as sovereign does not imply that He is a master without compassion. Why must we assume that He insists on His "owner's rights" through untold suffering and to the bitter end? How indeed can we know that "such is His Exalted Will?" ... God's greatness could rather be reflected in depth of compassion, allowing suicide which shortens terminal suffering.[45]

A few thinkers in each tradition are even more skeptical of any claims that continued life reflects God's will. For Catholic theologian Daniel Maguire,

The question now arising is whether, in certain circumstances, we may intervene creatively to achieve death by choice or whether mortal man must in all cases await the good pleasure of biochemical and organic factors and allow these to determine the time and manner of his demise. In more religious language, can the will of God regarding a person's death be manifested only through the collapse of sick or wounded organs or could it also be discovered through the sensitivities and reasonings of moral men?[46]

For Reform rabbi Alvin Reines, "every person is the ultimate owner of her/himself, with the moral right, consequently, to do with her/his mind or body that which she/he chooses to do. . . . A Reform Jew has a moral right to commit suicide . . . [and] . . . can give another person the moral right to take [his or her] life."[47]

A common theme in challenges to traditional prohibitions against euthanasia is that these rules are generally valuable but could have exceptions. In particular, euthanasia proponents challenge the distinction between active euthanasia and passive forgoing of treatment. Thinkers argue that although there is some value in this distinction it is not absolute, and active killing is not absolutely prohibited.[48] For Jewish and Catholic thinkers alike, love of neighbor in a specific situation might require an exception to a rule against euthanasia.[49] Because an absolute rule against euthanasia cannot be proven, individuals should have the right to follow their conscience.[50]

Some opponents of euthanasia respond that there simply *are* absolute rules, including that prohibiting euthanasia. Others argue that although exceptions to rules are possible, they must be prudential and carefully tailored to meet the needs of a pressing value. According to the Reform responsum, "As Reform Jews, of course, we consider our-selves free to ascribe 'new' Jewish meanings to our texts, to depart from tradition when we think it necessary to secure an essential religious or moral value. In this case, though, we fail to see why we should do so. We see no good reason, first of all, to abandon the traditional Jewish teaching concerning the inestimable value of human life."[51] McCormick reflects a similar approach in his response to Maguire.

> We build exception-clauses into concrete behavioral norms when we see clearly that a higher human value is being compromised, or at least can be, by failure to allow for exceptions. To do this with intel-lectual rigor and satisfaction, it seems that we must grasp clearly two things: the reason why the behavioral norm is generally valid in the first place, and the particular conflicting value that puts a limit on this validity. . . . Perhaps a concrete prohibition like the one in ques-tion cannot be "proved" [absolutely in the manner of geometry], but it might well be the conclusion of prudence in the face of dangers too momentous to allow the matter to the uncertainties and vulnerabil-ities of individual decisions.[52]

In response to warnings about the risks of abuse, proponents of euthanasia typically state that one simply must be careful in making case-by-case judgments that euthanasia is appropriate. Similarly, in response to policy concerns regarding the spread of institutionalized killing, proponents counsel that society must work carefully to develop appropriate safeguards.

There may be a somewhat greater reluctance among Jewish writ-ers than among Catholic writers to endorse policy changes legalizing euthanasia. Although Zohar notes theoretical reasons that could sup-port euthanasia, he asserts that the dangers of expanded killing raise "serious concerns," and the advisability of authorizing euthanasia as a practice requires further investigation. Knobel expresses profound concern with changing societal norms and voices support for decrim-inalization rather than legalization, characterizing suicide or euthana-sia as "an act not valid in the first instance but valid after the fact."[53] Thus, many Jewish writers who see themselves as supporting euthana-sia develop policy recommendations that are generally similar to those of Catholic writer Bresnahan, who presents himself as rejecting physician-assisted suicide. For Bresnahan, "some forms of legal toleration must be accorded to those who sincerely believe that self-killing is a morally justified . . . way for them to deal with the dying process, and who claim the right to help from like-minded persons," although "effective restraints must be imposed on such legally permitted practice of the inflicted death option."[54]

Only a few thinkers in each tradition reject these policy considerations as insignificant. For Reines, state laws against suicide or euthanasia either reflect a view that the political community is superior to and effectively "owns" the individual or represent the imposition of one religious belief on nonbelievers who may disagree. Reines summarily rejects such laws, without addressing policy risks that might be involved.[55] Maguire acknowledges potential problems, but it is clear to him that these problems will be resolved to allow euthanasia. An individual patient should be aware of personal and financial forces that might be inappropriately influencing a decision to end life and "beware lest he is yielding to societal pressures to measure human dignity in terms of utility." Policy concerns should be considered in developing legal safeguards, but Maguire assumes that these safeguards can be developed and euthanasia should be legalized. Doubting the possibility of adequate legal safeguards "is the hackneyed argument of the legal rigorist, who feels that only frozen categories are safe," Maguire writes. "It is the argument that has been thrown against the legalization of every advance of human freedom in the history of mores and laws."[56]

Although Catholic and Jewish writings supporting the moral validity of euthanasia share many elements, they also reveal a few differences. Jewish arguments, much more than Catholic arguments, tend to deal with traditional texts that are quoted at length and carefully analyzed.[57] Catholic writers supporting euthanasia (like Catholic writers who oppose it) place far more emphasis than their Jewish counterparts on a normative model of the good death. For example, Farley writes, "Is it not conceivable that profound 'acceptance' of death, acknowledgment of an ending that is indeed God's will, can be expressed through action as well as through passion?" In developing this view, she analyzes not texts but the experience and theology of the sacrament of communion.[58]

Conclusion

This brief survey of Jewish and Catholic writings on euthanasia suggests that there are impressive convergences between the two traditions. Theologians in these traditions frame the issues in similar ways and identify similar sets of specific concerns, often using virtually identical language. Moreover, a spectrum of responses on euthanasia and assisted suicide emerges in each faith community. On the whole, Jewish writers exhibit a greater tendency to cite legal (halakhic) precedent and other texts from the tradition. This approach accords with general characteristics of Jewish ethics and Judaism more broadly.[59] There also is a somewhat greater emphasis on policy implications of the law and perhaps a somewhat greater caution regarding proposed safeguards and reluctance to endorse legal change. This caution may correspond with the Jewish tradition's appreciation for the central role of law in shaping communal and personal life. It also may reflect the power of the Holocaust in Jewish thinking and consequently sensitivity to the dangers of institutionalized killing.[60]

Catholic writers exhibit a greater tendency to write in terms of teleology in general and the normative model of a good death in particular. This emphasis accords with the stronger role of teleology in Catholic ethics.[61] It also reflects the central role of Christ's death on the cross as a model for Catholic (and more generally Christian) faith and practice. Although Judaism has important narratives of martyrs who were willing to die for the sanctification of God's name, these models do not have the centrality and dominant role of Christ's passion.

In the conclusion to this book I undertake a fuller analysis of similarities between Jewish and Catholic writers on euthanasia and other issues, but I offer a few preliminary suggestions here. One is that shared values of the two faith traditions, rooted in the Hebrew Bible, do play a decisive role in the development of normative views. Judaism classically focuses on the study of texts and tradition and Catholicism on natural law and reason. The difference is not absolute, however, because all approaches within Judaism utilize reason, and Catholic reasoning is explicitly and implicitly shaped by tradition. In addition, these differences in methodology may provide different ways to draw on a similar core of values. The influence of these core values helps to explain the similarities in results—for euthanasia, both the tendency among Jewish and Catholic authorities to oppose these practices and the concerns and arguments presented by opponents and proponents.

More ambitiously, Jewish and Catholic thinkers may largely agree on certain ethical conclusions because they are true. As intersubjective agreement generally is understood as a warrant for objectivity (or its equivalent), agreement among views from different faith traditions may help to warrant these considerations as true for humans generally. Awareness of these overlapping concerns may help us in considering the role of religious voices in public ethics, identifying shared human values with what one hopes are special sensitivities to norms such as the dignity and worth of all human persons.[62]

Awareness of differing tendencies is important as well—with regard to euthanasia as well as other issues on which differences are more pronounced. At minimum, dialogue with a tradition that at once differs from and shares much with one's own could play a heuristic role, helping one to envision new possibilities or become sensitive to concerns that arise from shared values. Consideration of the insights of another tradition can afford a perspective that leads to each tradition being challenged and enriched. For example, Catholic writings on the spirituality of dying may help Jewish thinkers reappropriate and develop reflections along these lines within Judaism. Even where differences persist, awareness may lead to appreciation of the distinctive contributions of one's own faith tradition and the richness of human religious thought.

Notes

1. Thomas Aquinas, *Summa Theologiae [ST]* II-II, 64, 5, volume 38 of Blackfriars edition, trans. Marcus Lefébure (New York: McGraw-Hill and London: Eyre and Spottiswoode, 1975), 30–37; Benedict M. Ashley and Kevin D. O'Rourke, *Health Care Ethics: A Theological Analysis*, 4th ed. (Washington, D.C.: Georgetown University Press, 1997), 415–16. As I discuss, advocates of euthanasia may acknowledge this threefold set of concerns, even while they argue for exceptions in certain cases; see Margaret Farley, "Issues in Contemporary Christian Ethics: The Choice of Death in a Medical Context," presentation at Santa Clara University, May 1995; published as *The Santa Clara Lectures* 1, 3 (Santa Clara, Calif.: Santa Clara University, 1995).

2. Aquinas, *ST*; Yehiel M. Tuchinski, *Gesher Haḥayyim* (Jerusalem: Solomon, 1960), 1:269. Tuchinski also presents suicide as an even more blatant rejection of divine sovereignty than murder.

3. Ashley and O'Rourke, *Health Care Ethics*, 412; Elliot N. Dorff, "Physician-Assisted Suicide and Euthanasia," in *Life and Death Responsibilities in Jewish Biomedical Ethics*, ed. Aaron L. Mackler (New York: Jewish Theological Seminary of America, Finkelstein Institute, 2000), 409–10; J. David Bleich, *Judaism and Healing* (New York: Ktav, 1981), 158–61; Tuchinski, *Gesher Haḥayyim*, 270–73. Tuchinski also notes the possibility that the person who committed suicide repented his or her act in the final moments of life.

4. *Origins* 24 (1994): 458.

5. Aquinas, *ST* II-II, 64, 5, pp. 32–33; Eliezer Yehudah Waldenberg, *Ramat Raḥel*, no. 29, in *Tzitz Eliezer* (Jerusalem: n.p., 1985), 5:38–39.

6. John J. Paris, "Autonomy and Physician-Assisted Suicide," *America* 176, no. 17 (1997): 13.

7. Dorff, "Physician-Assisted Suicide and Euthanasia," 415.

8. Congregation for the Doctrine of the Faith, "Declaration on Euthanasia," *Origins* 10 (1980): 155.

9. Immanuel Jakobovits, *Jewish Medical Ethics*, rev. ed. (New York: Bloch, 1975), 275.

10. Aquinas, *ST* II-II, 64, 5, p. 35

11. Bleich, *Judaism and Healing*, 136.

12. Jean deBlois and Kevin D. O'Rourke, "Issues at the End of Life," *Health Progress* 76, no. 6 (1995): 25. See similarly Oregon and Washington Bishops, "Living and Dying Well," *Origins* 21 (1991): 347.

13. Dorff, "Physician-Assisted Suicide and Euthanasia," 416. Similarly Bleich, *Judaism and Healing*, 136: "As long as man is yet endowed with a spark of life—as defined by God's eternal law—man dare not presume to hasten death, no matter how hopeless or meaningless continued existence may appear in the eye of a mortal perceiver."

14. *Evangelium Vitae: The Gospel of Life [EV]* (Washington, D.C.: United States Catholic Conference, 1995), n. 66, p. 121.

15. "On the Treatment of the Terminally Ill," in *Teshuvot for the Nineties: Reform Judaism's Answers to Today's Dilemmas*, ed. W. Gunther Plaut and Mark Washofsky (New York: Central Conference of American Rabbis, 1997), 341.

16. *EV*, n. 64, pp. 115–16.

17. Bernard Häring, *Medical Ethics*, ed. Gabrielle L. Jean (Notre Dame, Ind.: Fides, 1973), 148.

18. Dorff, "Physician-Assisted Suicide and Euthanasia," 414.

19. Richard McCormick, "Technology, the Consistent Ethic, and Assisted Suicide," *Origins* 25 (1995): 460.

20. Dorff, "Physician-Assisted Suicide and Euthanasia," 415.

21. *EV* n. 66, p. 121; McCormick, "Technology, the Consistent Ethic, and Assisted Suicide," 460. Likewise, Ashley and O'Rourke, *Health Care Ethics,* 416, write, "When persons freely choose to die and ask to be killed, they are not only committing the crime of suicide but also compounding it by making another a partner in the crime. To yield to such a request is false compassion. . . . To have true compassion for the person who has made such a decision is to realize that the person feels hopeless, alienated from community, and doubtful of God's love. Mercy entails staying by such a person's side and through friendship helping him or her to recover hope."

22. Dorff, "Physician-Assisted Suicide and Euthanasia," 427. According to the Reform responsum ("Treatment of the Terminally Ill," 343), "when we define 'compassion' so as to include the killing of human beings, we have transgressed the most elemental of Jewish moral standards and the most basic teachings of Jewish tradition as we understand it."

23. McCormick, "Technology, the Consistent Ethic, and Assisted Suicide," 461, 463; U.S. Conference of Catholic Bishops, "Ethical and Religious Directives for Catholic Health Care Services," 459, n. 61; Dorff, "Physician-Assisted Suicide and Euthanasia," 419–20. See also Oregon and Washington Bishops, "Living and Dying Well," 351.

24. Congregation for the Doctrine of the Faith, "Declaration on Euthanasia," 156. Similarly *EV*, n. 67, p. 123.

25. Richard A. McCormick, *Notes on Moral Theology 1965–1980* (Washington, D.C.: University Press of America, 1981), 604, quoting *On Dying Well* (London: Church Information Office, 1975).

26. "Treatment of the Terminally Ill," 341; emphasis in original.

27. Bleich, *Judaism and Healing;* Waldenberg, *Ramat Raḥel,* no. 29; see also chapter 4.

28. Jakobovits, *Jewish Medical Ethics.*

29. Dorff, "Physician-Assisted Suicide and Euthanasia," 420; similarly "Treatment of the Terminally Ill," 344–52.

30. Congregation for the Doctrine of the Faith, "Declaration on Euthanasia," 156; *EV*, n. 65, p. 117.

31. Paris, "Autonomy and Physician-Assisted Suicide," 12; similarly McCormick, "Technology, the Consistent Ethic, and Assisted Suicide," 462. According to the bishops' "Ethical and Religious Directives," "two extremes are avoided: on the one hand, an insistence on useless or burdensome technology even when a patient may legitimately wish to forgo it and, on the

other hand, the withdrawal of technology with the intention of causing death" (458).

32. James F. Bresnahan, "Observations on the Rejection of Physician-Assisted Suicide: A Roman Catholic Perspective," *Christian Bioethics* 1 (1995): 257–61.

33. Häring, *Medical Ethics*, 148–49; similarly McCormick, *Notes on Moral Theology*. Both explicitly refer to the expansion of institutionalized killing under the Nazis (Häring, 144; McCormick, 443).

34. Dorff, "Physician-Assisted Suicide and Euthanasia," 418; emphasis in original.

35. "Treatment of the Terminally Ill," 342–43. Other writers, such as Waldenberg, note such policy concerns as supplementary to their basic opposition to the inherent wrongness of euthanasia.

36. McCormick, *Notes on Moral Theology*, 436; similarly 446.

37. Bresnahan, "Observations on the Rejection of Physician-Assisted Suicide," 257; Häring, *Medical Ethics*, 149.

38. Farley, "Issues in Contemporary Christian Ethics," 17.

39. Peter Knobel, "Suicide, Assisted Suicide, Active Euthanasia: A Halakhic Inquiry," in *Death and Euthanasia in Jewish Law: Essays and Responsa*, ed. Walter Jacob and Moshe Zemer (Pittsburgh: Rodef Shalom Press, 1995), 48.

40. Byron Sherwin, "A View of Euthanasia," in *Contemporary Jewish Ethics and Morality*, ed. Elliot N. Dorff and Louis E. Newman (New York: Oxford University Press, 1995), 365; Farley, "Issues in Contemporary Christian Ethics," 1–2.

41. Noam J. Zohar, *Alternatives in Jewish Bioethics* (Albany: State University of New York Press, 1997), 54.

42. Sherwin, "A View of Euthanasia," 370.

43. Farley, "Issues in Contemporary Christian Ethics," 5; Knobel, "Suicide, Assisted Suicide, Active Euthanasia," 41–42. As this quotation suggests, Knobel cites the views of secular ethicist Dan Brock several times in his paper.

44. Charles E. Curran, *Politics, Medicine, and Christian Ethics: A Dialogue with Paul Ramsey* (Philadelphia: Fortress, 1973), 161–62; see similarly Farley, "Issues in Contemporary Christian Ethics," 13.

45. Zohar, *Alternatives in Jewish Bioethics*, 56–58.

46. Daniel Maguire, "The Freedom to Die," *Commonweal* 96 (1972): 424.

47. Alvin J. Reines, "Reform Judaism, Bioethics, and Abortion," *Journal of Reform Judaism* 37 (1990): 44–45. For Reines, the only plausible basis for a limitation on suicide would be a belief that a "theistic God has commanded through an inerrant revelation that the human person is prohibited

from destroying that which ultimately belongs to Him, namely, the human person's life, and has given to the Orthodox Jewish rabbinate (if one is an Orthodox Jew) or to the Roman Catholic hierarchy (if one is Roman Catholic) the right to enforce His prohibition over their communities" (48).

48. Farley, "Issues in Contemporary Christian Ethics," 14, 7–11; Maguire, "The Freedom to Die"; Knobel, "Suicide, Assisted Suicide, Active Euthanasia."

49. Daniel C. Maguire, "A Catholic View of Mercy Killing," in *Beneficent Euthanasia*, ed. Marvin Kohl (Buffalo, N.Y.: Prometheus, 1975), 37–38; Leonard Kravitz, "Euthanasia," in *Death and Euthanasia in Jewish Law*, 22.

50. Maguire, "The Freedom to Die," 426; Reines, "Reform Judaism, Bioethics, and Abortion."

51. "Treatment of the Terminally Ill," 340. Concerns also are expressed regarding the expansion of killing and potential abuse, as noted above. In a related context (351–52), the Reform writers parallel McCormick in acknowledging potential uncertainty in reaching moral judgments but asserting that one nevertheless must seek the most strongly warranted conclusion. "Our task is to determine the best answer, the one that most closely corresponds to our understanding of the tradition as a whole. That search must be conducted by means of analysis, interpretation, and argument. Its outcome will never enjoy the finality of the solution to a mathematical equation; its conclusions will be subject to challenge and critique. Yet this is no reason to shrink from moral argument; it means rather that we have no choice but to enter the fray, to confront difficult cases, and to do the best we can."

52. McCormick, *Notes on Moral Theology*, 442–43.

53. Zohar, *Alternatives in Jewish Bioethics*, 61–62; Knobel, "Suicide, Assisted Suicide, Active Euthanasia," 46. Knobel (27) warns, "In challenging established societal norms which seek to protect individual human life, one could begin a process which radically alters the way in which society treats the weak and the vulnerable. If we propose an attitude shift in the 'hard cases' do we change the attitude of individuals and society so as to encourage suicide and lead from a situation where people willingly waive their right not to be killed, under severely limited circumstances, to involuntary active euthanasia based on social worth?" Sherwin does not address the issue of legalization; he presents himself as developing a minority position in the tradition that "individuals whose last days are overwhelmed with unbearable agony, should be able to advocate and to practice euthanasia without feeling that they are criminals, without being burdened with great guilt for actions that they consider merciful, without feeling that they have transgressed divine and human laws, and without feeling that they have rejected the teachings of the Jewish tradition"; "A View of Euthanasia," 376.

54. Bresnahan, "Observations on the Rejection of Physician-Assisted Suicide," 273.

55. Reines, "Reform Judaism, Bioethics, and Abortion," 48–51.

56. Maguire, "The Freedom to Die," 426; "Catholic View," 39.

57. E.g., Zohar, *Alternatives in Jewish Bioethics;* Sherwin, "A View of Euthanasia"; Knobel, "Suicide, Assisted Suicide, Active Euthanasia."

58. Farley, "Issues in Contemporary Christian Ethics," 13. Catholic writers such as Farley often are more inclined to justify euthanasia on the basis of a low "quality of life" (5). This approach accords with a greater willingness among Catholic than Jewish writers to explicitly invoke quality of life in forgoing life-sustaining treatment (see chapter 4).

59. See discussion in chapter 2.

60. See Conclusion for further discussion.

61. See discussion in chapter 1.

62. See, e.g., Lisa Sowle Cahill, "Can Theology Have a Role in 'Public' Bioethical Discourse?" *Hastings Center Report* 20, no. 4 (1990, suppl.): 10–14, and discussion in Conclusion.

Chapter 4

Treatment Decisions Near the End of Life

TREATMENT DECISIONS NEAR THE END OF LIFE ARE AMONG the most common—and most wrenching—issues in bioethics. In countries such as the United States, most deaths are accompanied by decisions about whether to forgo life-sustaining treatment. These situations include dramatic decisions to terminally wean a patient from a respirator, controversial decisions to forgo artificial nutrition and hydration, and simple and sometimes implicit decisions not to try yet another round of chemotherapy. Choices about forgoing treatment can be informed by values and precedents of traditional discourse. They have generated extensive discussion in Jewish and Catholic bioethics.

Discerning treatment decisions near the end of life involves central values of each tradition in powerful but often ambiguous ways. Respect for divine sovereignty and the responsibilities of stewardship could support continuing life-sustaining treatment, avoiding what might be regarded as a decision against life; yet at some point respect for divine sovereignty may require letting go and accepting the inevitable end of mortal life. Values such as love of neighbor and human dignity could support either continuing treatment or allowing a patient to die.

Judaism and Roman Catholicism share a commitment to the value of life and the responsibility to provide healing to persons in need. Life is understood to be a gift entrusted to human persons by a loving and beneficent Creator, the author and sustainer of life. Accordingly, people are responsible to preserve life and health and to pursue effective and beneficial medical treatment. Both traditions have long opposed active euthanasia, assisted suicide, and suicide, and most authorities today continue this opposition. The two traditions agree that patients have some range of autonomous choice but that, at least as a moral matter, this range is constrained by objective moral limits. For patients who are dying or suffering, the extent of the responsibility to provide and accept care becomes a pressing question. The question is framed by Catholic ethicist Gerald Kelly: "How much does God demand that I do in order to preserve this life which belongs to God and of which I am only a steward?"[1]

In addressing this question, each tradition draws on its understanding of reason and human experience—an understanding shaped by authoritative texts of the tradition. In Jewish ethics, citation and interpretation of traditional texts is prevalent in addressing all issues. In the Catholic tradition, discussion of authoritative texts is more prominent on end-of-life issues than on many others. Catholic authors contest the implications of Francisco de Vitoria's sixteenth-century analysis of the obligation to eat and receive medical treatment or the significance of Pope Pius XII's understanding of ordinary and extraordinary treatment.[2] This proliferation of rival interpretations partly reflects centuries of wrestling with these concerns. Magisterial statements on this issue also have tended to be nuanced or ambiguous, leaving room for competing views (to a much greater degree than pronouncements on euthanasia, abortion, or reproductive technologies).

In this chapter I begin by considering some of the most influential texts shaping deliberation in the Catholic and Jewish traditions. I examine the diverse ways in which thinkers in each tradition conceptualize the issues involved in end-of-life decisions and formulate practical guidelines. Many thinkers in each tradition agree that treatments may be forgone when they become inappropriate—but never as a way to seek death.[3] I survey the spectrum of positions taken on end-of-life decisions in each tradition, noting the extensive overlap of the spectra and the tendency of Catholic thinkers to be somewhat more liberal on these issues—more ready to forgo life-sustaining treatment. I discuss four general approaches: maintaining all life-sustaining treatment; allowing forgoing of treatment that is therapeutically ineffective or intrinsically burdensome, especially for dying patients; allowing forgoing of treatment when burdens exceed benefits (construing these terms broadly); and authorizing forgoing of treatment when it would fail to enhance the patient's ability to pursue life's purpose.

Authoritative Texts

In the Catholic tradition, significant discussion regarding the extent of the obligation to preserve one's life began to develop in the sixteenth century. Francisco de Vitoria argued that although an individual has an obligation to sustain his own life by means of food, there are limits to this obligation. In general, "it is licit to eat common and regular foods." An individual would not be required to eat special foods, such as poultry, even if these were available and would extend his life—just as individuals are not obligated to move so that they can live in the most healthful place. Furthermore, an individual would not be obligated to eat even commonly available food if doing so would require great effort or entail unusual burdens. "If a sick man can take food or nourishment with some hope of life, he is held to take the food, as he would be held to give it to one who is sick. . . . If the depression of the spirit is so low and there is present such consternation in the appetitive power that only with the greatest of effort and as though by means of certain torture, can the sick man take food, right away that is reckoned a certain impossibility, and therefore he is excused, at least from mortal sin, especially where there is little hope of life, or none at all." Vitoria sharply distinguishes between an absolute prohibition against killing and a more limited positive obligation to support life. "It is one thing not to protect life and it is another to destroy it: for man is not always held to the first and it is enough that he perform that by which regularly a man can live: if a sick man could not have a drug except by giving over his whole means of subsistence, I do not think he would be bound to do so." The obligation to take medicine allows for additional flexibility because food is more clearly a natural means intended for the conservation of life. In principle, if one were certain to live if one took a drug, and certain to die otherwise, one would be obligated to take the drug; in practice, "this rarely can be certain," so medicine is optional.[4]

In the seventeenth century, Cardinal Juan de Lugo addressed the extent and limit of the obligation to sustain one's life. "A man must guard his life by ordinary means against dangers and death coming from natural causes . . . because the one who neglects the ordinary means seems to neglect his life and therefore to act negligently in the administration of it, and he who does not employ the ordinary means which nature has provided for the ordinary conservation of life is considered morally to will his death." On the other hand, difficult and extraordinary means are not obligatory, and one who forgoes these means is not considered to will death. For example, a patient must undergo mutilating surgery "when the doctors judge it necessary, and when it can happen without intense pain; not, if it is accompanied by very bitter pain; because a man is not bound to employ extraordinary and difficult means to conserve his life." Further, actions that would prolong life only briefly are not obligatory. If a man is condemned to being burned to death and has enough water to extinguish the fire which would then be relit, "he would not be held to use this means to conserve his life for such a brief time because the obligation of conserving life by ordinary means is not an obligation of using means for such a brief conservation—which is morally considered nothing at all."[5]

De Lugo's distinction between "ordinary" and "extraordinary" means and his concern with the will or intention of the agent have remained central in Catholic discussion until the present time. In 1958 Gerald Kelly provided what have become classic definitions:

> *Ordinary* means of preserving life are all medicines, treatments, and operations, which offer a reasonable hope of benefit for the patient and which can be obtained and used without excessive expense, pain, or other inconvenience. . . . In contradistinction to ordinary are *extraordinary* means of preserving life. By these we mean all medicines, treatments, and operations, which cannot be obtained or used without excessive expense, pain, or other inconvenience, or which, if used, would not offer a reasonable hope of benefit.[6]

Pope Pius XII had addressed this issue a year previously, stating that there is an obligation

> in case of serious illness to take the necessary treatment for the preservation of life and health. . . . But normally one is held to use only ordinary means—according to circumstances of persons, places, times, and culture—that is to say, means that do not involve any grave burden for oneself or another. A more strict obligation would be too burdensome for most men and would render the attainment of the higher, more important good too difficult. Life, health, all temporal activities are in fact subordinated to spiritual ends.

More aggressive or burdensome treatment would not be required—but would remain permitted to the patient, "as long as he does not fail in some more serious duty."[7]

A second influential magisterial statement was the "Declaration on Euthanasia" issued in 1980 by the Congregation for the Doctrine of the Faith (see chapter 3). This document condemns euthanasia—understood as "an action or an omission which of itself or by intention causes death, in order that all suffering may in this way be eliminated." Euthanasia is characterized both in terms of "the intention of the will" and "the methods used." Yet although one has a duty to seek appropriate ("proportionate") health care, one is not obliged to use "extraordinary," or "disproportionate," means. Specifically, it is permissible

> to make do with the normal means that medicine can offer. Therefore one cannot impose on anyone the obligation to have recourse to a technique which is already in use but which carries a risk or is burdensome. Such a refusal is not the equivalent of suicide; on the contrary, it should be considered as an acceptance of the human condition, or a wish to avoid the application of a medical procedure disproportionate to the results that can be expected, or a desire not to impose excessive expense on the family or the community.

In addition, "when inevitable death is imminent in spite of the means used, it is permitted in conscience to take the decision to refuse forms of treatment that would only secure a precarious and burdensome prolongation of life, so long as the normal care due to the sick person in similar cases is not interrupted." Furthermore, "Life is a gift of God, and on the other hand, death is unavoidable; it is necessary therefore that we, without in any way hastening the hour of death, should be able to accept it with full responsibility and dignity."[8]

Jewish discussions of treatment decisions near the end of life reflect the tradition's general imperative to heal and save life, as noted in the Introduction. Whereas for Vitoria medicine is generally encouraged but not obligatory, it is very much obligatory in the legal code of his contemporary, Joseph Karo—the *Shulḥan Arukh*. "The Torah gave permission for the physician to heal. That is a mitzvah [commandment], and is in the category of saving life [*pikuaḥ nefesh*]. If the physician abstains from healing, he is one who sheds blood." According to the Talmud and later Jewish authorities, the imperative to save life is virtually always decisive, superseding competing considerations. If a building collapses on the Sabbath, the debris must be cleared immediately even though this activity would violate the observance of the holy day, even if it is uncertain whether any person is trapped or whether anyone remains alive. Debris must be cleared even if it is obvious that a victim could live only an hour or two because that short extension of life is precious.[9] Whereas the Catholic tradition provides de Lugo's precedent of a man being burned—suggesting that brief prolongation of life is not worth pursuing—the Talmud's ruling indicates that brief prolongation of life is valuable: enough to justify violation of the legal requirements of the Sabbath.[10]

The central Jewish text for deliberating about treatment decisions near the end of life is found in Karo's *Shulḥan Arukh*. "A *goseis* [imminently dying patient] is considered as alive in all respects. . . . One does not close his eyes until his soul departs. Anyone who closes the eyes [of the *goseis*] at the moment of the soul's departure is considered as one who has shed blood."[11] The standard text of the *Shulḥan Arukh* continues with the interspersed commentary (*Mapah*) of Moses Isserles.

> Thus, it is forbidden to cause the dying person to die more quickly. For example, if one is a *goseis* for a long time and is unable to expire, it is forbidden to remove the pillow or mattress from underneath him, . . . and one does not move him from his place. However, if there is something causing a hindrance to the soul's departure, such as if there is a noise near the house such as a woodchopper, or if there is salt on his tongue, and these are delaying the departure of the soul, it is permitted to remove them—this is not a [significant] action, but the removal of an impediment.[12]

Jewish writers have been influenced by narratives of the aggadah in addition to these halakhic rulings. Prominent among these narratives is the Talmud's account of the martyrdom of Rabbi Ḥanina ben Teradyon. The Roman authorities condemned him to death by fire and placed woolen tufts soaked in water on his heart, "so that his soul would not depart quickly." His students called on him to open his mouth so that the flames would enter, speeding death. Rabbi Ḥanina refused, replying, "It is better that He who gave my soul should take it, and a man should not injure himself." When the executioner offered to increase the fire and remove the woolen tufts, however, Rabbi Ḥanina agreed.[13]

These texts have been central to Jewish deliberations about end-of-life decisions and generally are considered to support some scope for allowing death to occur, while prohibiting active killing and the hastening of death. The texts are ambiguous, however, and the implications of these texts for contemporary health care are subject to debate. Is the *goseis* from whom interventions may be removed one who is certain to die within seventy-two hours or a terminally ill patient who may have months to live? May medical interventions be forgone, or only folk remedies of questionable effectiveness? For some Jewish thinkers, rulings about woodchoppers and stories of Roman executioners are too distant from today's hospitals to be relevant; for others, these texts (like De Lugo's discussion of a burning man with limited water) provide valuable paradigm cases that concretize fundamental principles of the tradition.[14]

Approaches to Treatment Decisions: Maintaining All Life-Sustaining Treatment

Influenced by the texts and values of their traditions, Jewish and Catholic writers express a wide variety of views on treatment decisions near the end of life. Jewish and Catholic positions on these issues represent overlapping spectra, with the Jewish spectrum extending somewhat to the right—expressing greater reluctance to forgo medical interventions. Four general approaches are evident. First, among some Orthodox Jewish authorities life-sustaining treatments must be continued in virtually all cases, including those involving dying patients. A second approach would agree with the first that life is intrinsically beneficial and death may never be sought. Nevertheless, some life-sustaining measures may be forgone for a terminally ill patient if these measures entail intrinsic burdens or will not offer therapeutic benefit, especially if a patient is imminently dying. Many Jewish thinkers, as well as some Catholic writers, articulate this view. A third approach is similar but takes a broader view of benefits and burdens, authorizing a broader range of decisions to forgo treatment. This approach has been dominant in the Roman Catholic tradition and appears among some Jewish thinkers as well. A final set of views, which is common among many Catholic thinkers, gives great weight to the patient's quality of life and ability to pursue the purpose of life; life-sustaining interventions are pointless when that ability is absent.

Some thinkers in each tradition emphasize the intrinsic benefit of continued life, supporting the provision of life-sustaining treatment. For some Orthodox Jewish writers, the obligation to maintain life-sustaining treatment is almost absolute. Immanuel Jakobovits speaks of "Judaism's attribution of *infinite* value to human life. Infinity being indivisible, any fraction of life, however limited its expectancy or its health, remains equally infinite in value." Similarly, J. David Bleich argues—on the basis of leniencies regarding ritual prohibitions in order to preserve life—that "not only is every human life of infinite value but every moment of human life is of infinite value." Humans are charged with the obligation to sustain life, and any continuation of life, even when it is marked by suffering, is esteemed as a benefit for the patient.[15] Accordingly, some Orthodox Jewish authorities restrict the forgoing of treatment to very narrow circumstances. For some, the permission to forgo interventions for a *goseis* applies only if death is certain within seventy-two hours or if the patient is brain dead. Furthermore, the interventions that may licitly be forgone may be limited to folk remedies of questionable effectiveness or medical interventions that are futile in the sense of having no physiological effect. Even these thinkers note that treatments often entail risk or may be only questionably effective, allowing some room for decisions about providing treatment. Nevertheless, in virtually all circumstances, all treatment that is effective in prolonging life must be provided.[16]

Avoiding Prolongation of Dying and Forgoing Therapeutically Ineffective Treatment

Other thinkers, while agreeing on the intrinsic goodness of life, allow a greater scope for decisions to forgo life-sustaining treatment. Such forgoing of treatment is accepted most broadly for patients who are dying and for treatment that directly imposes significant burdens. Among Jewish thinkers, this view is supported textually by an expanded reading of the paradigm of removing hindrances to dying from the *goseis*. Against the claim that *goseis* applies only in the last three days of life, writers note passages in rabbinic literature suggesting that some individuals in this condition live more than three or four days. Indeed, Isserles writes of an individual who is a *goseis* for a long time. Some thinkers also suggest that whereas in earlier centuries a *goseis* would die quickly, modern technology can prolong the dying state. Conservative writer Avram Reisner argues that *goseis* refers "to all those who have been diagnosed as imminently dying," or to all who are terminally ill. For Reisner and others, the paradigm of removing factors that delay the natural dying process is decisive. This model allows for the forgoing of life-sustaining treatment in some cases, without compromising the intrinsic value of life and the decisive obligation to save life. "The halakhic sources ask us to define the distinction between extending life—any life, not just 'quality life,' for even the smallest duration—and prolonging the process of dying."[17]

Some Orthodox authorities, such as Shlomo Auerbach, share views similar to those described in the preceding section—that prolonging life for each additional moment would be valuable—but judge that this standard is not always obligatory. Treatments that entail suffering need not be imposed on a patient who refuses them, though ideally the patient would be persuaded to accept these interventions because of the value of even one hour of life. Other writers claim that artificially prolonging the dying process is undesirable—and indeed forbidden.[18] Numerous Orthodox authorities permit forgoing some treatments by characterizing them as hindrances to the dying process.[19] Conservative thinker David Feldman writes, "A clear distinction is thus implied between the deliberate termination of life and the removal of means that artificially prolong the process of death. . . . While physicians, then, may not disconnect life-support systems where they shorten life thereby, they may do so to shorten the dying process." (Feldman acknowledges that because "it is difficult to tell the difference between shortening life and death, the principle is a moral one more than a practical one.")[20] A model advance directive from the Reform movement offers a similar understanding of treatment decisions near the end of life. "Jewish tradition affirms the sanctity of life. Yet, when there is no hope for the patient and death is certain, one should not hasten his death, but at the same time, one should not prolong his death throes but permit him to die in peace."[21]

Several Jewish thinkers frame the issue as determining the scope of the obligation to heal and receive medical treatment. The question then is framed not as whether forgoing treatment could be justified but as whether providing treatment could be compelled—thus shifting the burden of proof. Jakobovits writes that provision of health care is obligatory only when it is possible to restore a patient to health. Accordingly, he would allow a suffering, terminally ill cancer patient to forgo insulin because the insulin would not be effective in bringing health to the patient. For Jakobovits, a conflict between the value of life, on one hand, and human dignity and compassion on the other is irreconcilable. Accordingly, one should refrain from action (*shev v'al ta'aseh*) and not impose treatment.[22] Similarly, Moshe Feinstein rules that an intervention that would only prolong the dying process of a suffering patient should not be considered obligatory healing.[23] Gedaliah Aharon Rabinowitz and Mordecai Koenigsberg write that the obligation to rescue persons in need would not apply to interventions that would prolong the life of a permanently unconscious patient with no hope for recovery.[24] A responsum from the Reform movement articulates an approach that is generally similar to these Orthodox authorities: "Once a medical treatment ceases to be effective and beneficial it ceases to be 'medicine' as that practice is conceived by Jewish tradition. . . . Treatments which do not effect 'healing' are not *medicine* and thus are not required."[25]

Jewish thinkers apply these arguments to authorize the forgoing of life-sustaining interventions on the ground that they merely prolong the dying process or that they do not constitute obligatory healing. Some limit interventions that might be regarded as impediments. Many Orthodox authorities require that routine treatments—including oxygen and standard medications (as well as nutrition and hydration)—must be continued. One authority rules that treatments intended specifically to treat an incurable, terminal illness may be forgone.[26] This view is reflected in a law proposed by Israel's Steinberg Commission on the Care of the Terminally Ill Patient. The commission articulates a presumption that a patient would want to continue to live and hence to receive life-sustaining treatment; this presumption could be rebutted by the contemporaneous statement of a competent patient or an advance directive providing clear and convincing evidence for a patient without capacity. The commission argues that Israeli law generally should reflect the majority view of Orthodox decisors because this approach presents the best available compromise between the values of sanctity of life and of autonomy. Treatments for an incurable illness may be forgone, but routine treatments of oxygen and medications (as well as nutrition and hydration) should be provided. If a competent patient refuses routine measures, health care professionals should persuade the patient to accept these measures—but a persistent refusal should be respected, in part because coerced treatment could lead to harm. Because attempts at persuasion are impossible for an incapacitated patient, routine measures must be provided. Unless there is a clear indication of the patient's wishes, life-sustaining treatment may be forgone only in the final stage of terminal illness—when a patient is not expected to survive longer than two weeks, more than one vital system has failed, and the patient is suffering. Only in this stage would an advance directive to forgo routine care be effective.[27]

Conservative rabbi Reisner takes a somewhat less restrictive view, arguing that mechanical respirators and transfusions might be forgone as impediments for a dying patient. Any interventions that are of uncertain effectiveness or that entail risk are not obligatory. A dying patient may refuse these treatments as long as the intention is to avoid burdens and allow death to occur naturally. ("Refusing life-giving treatment with an eye to ending life [would be] tantamount to suicide.") However, "all nutrition and medication against illness—antibiotics, insulin, intravenous fluids, and so on—organic treatments whose effectiveness is well established and that have no significant attendant risk, cannot be classified as impediments to death. These should generally be continued as long as they are effective."[28]

Several Orthodox writers are more flexible regarding the types of treatments that might be regarded as hindrances and hence nonobligatory.[29] A model advance directive from the Orthodox Rabbinical Council of America allows a person to forgo most types of interventions in the event that he or she becomes terminally ill and unable to communicate; these interventions include antibiotics and blood transfusions, as well as major surgery, chemotherapy, mechanical breathing, cardiopulmonary resuscitation, and dialysis. Moshe D. Tendler and Fred Rosner write that "if a patient near death is in severe pain and no therapeutic protocol holds any hope for recovery, it may be proper to withhold any additional pharmacological or technological interventions so as to permit the natural ebbing of the life forces."[30]

Many Jewish writers distinguish artificial nutrition and hydration from medical treatment, arguing that nutrition and hydration generally cannot be regarded as mere hindrances to the dying process, or as optional interventions. Although many Orthodox authorities allow the forgoing of medication and most other treatments, these writers generally insist that artificial nutrition and hydration be continued. Nutrition and hydration, however provided, represent natural means to fulfill a universal need. Forgoing these measures would represent killing. The Rabbinical Council advance directive, which allows options for most treatments in case of terminal illness, specifies, "I direct that in all cases food and liquids be given."[31]

Conservative thinker Avram Reisner requires continuation of intravenous feedings under most circumstances when they would be effective in prolonging life because they impose little risk or discomfort. "To withhold them is effectively a decision to hasten the death of the patient affected, since death by dehydration is likely to precede death from the underlying disease." Feeding tubes, however, entail significant discomfort and risk. Thus, there is greater leeway for a patient to refuse these interventions, without necessarily having the intention of causing death.[32] Some Orthodox authorities allow the forgoing of intravenous as well as tube feedings in exceptional circumstances, in the case of a dying patient who experiences pain and suffering.[33]

The Reform responsum acknowledges arguments that artificial nutrition and hydration are medical interventions that may be forgone when they fail to provide healing and that these interventions represent the fulfillment of basic human needs. The responsum leans toward the latter position.

> Food and water, no matter how they are delivered, are the very staff of life . . . for the human being. They sustain us at every moment of our lives, in health as well as in illness. It is therefore not at all obvious that we should look upon these substances as "medicine" merely because they come to us in the form of a tube inserted by medical professionals. . . . We cannot overlook the fact that by removing them we are starving these human beings to death. We would therefore caution at the very least that the removal of artificial nutrition and hydration should never become a routine procedure. It is preferable that artificial feeding of terminal patients be maintained so that,

when death comes, it will not have come because we have caused it by starvation.

The responsum concludes, however, that because this argument is not certain, patients and families may follow their own conscience on this matter.[34]

Most Jewish writers who have addressed the issue of permanently unconscious patients include them in the category of the terminally ill, with similar restrictions and allowances for forgoing treatment. The Rabbinical Council advance directive generally allows the same treatment choices for patients "in an irreversible coma or a persistent vegetative state" as for those who are terminally ill (though it describes antibiotics and simple diagnostic tests as mandatory for permanent unconscious patients but optional for terminally ill patients).[35] Reisner asserts that patients in a persistent vegetative state are not dying. Although he would authorize forgoing of mechanical interventions such as respirators, he argues that it generally would be difficult to justify forgoing life-sustaining treatment (in particular, artificial nutrition and hydration) on the basis of risk or patient discomfort, so these measures must be continued.[36] One Orthodox source, however, understands a permanently unconscious patient to be in an extended *goseis* state and rules that there is no obligation to prolong this condition. Nutrition and hydration, as well as mechanical interventions and medicines, would constitute hindrances to the dying process that may be forgone.[37]

An additional complication arises for most Orthodox thinkers who rely on the approach that in some cases life-sustaining treatment cannot be proven obligatory (rather than claiming that forgoing can be justified). For many of these writers withdrawal of treatments, such as a respirator, is harder to fit into the "lack of action" paradigm. Removal of the respirator, in this view, could be regarded as causing the death of the patient. Thus, most Orthodox authorities do not authorize removal of a respirator from a patient who requires its assistance. Nevertheless, many would not require the respirator to be provided as long as the technical prohibition against withdrawal is not violated. For example, it might be suggested that the respirator be attached to a timer that will automatically shut off after some time if it is not reset. Some writers suggest that when a respirator is temporarily removed for routine care (e.g., suctioning of the lungs), it need not be reconnected—thus qualifying as a withholding rather than a withdrawal.[38] Israel's Steinberg Commission recommends that Israeli law should not allow the removal of a respirator when this action is likely to lead to death—even at the request of a competent patient—but notes the possibility of changing the forgoing of a respirator to a withholding of treatment by means of a timer.[39]

Some Orthodox authorities accept the removal of a respirator from a *goseis*. Rabbi Ḥayyim David Halevi argues that a respirator can become like the grain of salt that Isserles ruled could be removed from a *goseis*. Even if the respirator initially was used to prolong life in hope of a cure, it may become clear that it is only artificially prolonging the dying process of the *goseis* and hence may—and indeed should—be removed.[40] Conservative and Reform writers generally understand the withdrawal of treatment as equivalent to withholding. As expressed by Feldman, "At the outset, the physician should connect the support systems of respiration or circulation; he should not decline to do so on the grounds that this may be prolonging death. He must give the patient every chance for life. Having connected the systems conditionally, however, he may remove them if he then determines that their function was not prolongation of life but of death."[41]

Some Catholic positions resemble some of the foregoing Jewish approaches. A statement on nutrition and hydration by William E. May, Robert Barry, and others shares much with Reisner's views. The statement declares that "human bodily life is a great good." Although life-sustaining treatment may be forgone if it is useless or excessively burdensome, prolongation of life constitutes a benefit, and "remaining alive is never rightly regarded as a burden." Accordingly, artificial nutrition and hydration should be provided for permanently unconscious patients. These measures provide the benefit of continued life without significant risks or burdens to the patient, so a decision to forgo them in such cases in effect would be a choice to kill the patient by omission. "*If it is really useless or excessively burdensome* to provide someone with nutrition and hydration, then these means may rightly be withheld or withdrawn, *provided* that this omission does not carry out a proposal to end the person's life, but rather is chosen to avoid the useless effort or the excessive burden of continuing to provide the food and fluids."[42] There is some room for this judgment to be made for imminently dying patients—corresponding to the category of *goseis* and Reisner's approach of allowing natural death.

Catholic thinkers generally do not see a significant distinction between whether treatment can be shown to be obligatory and whether the forgoing of treatment can be shown to be justified. This attitude may be common in part because the Catholic tradition affords greater resources for justifying forgoing of treatment as extraordinary. This approach also could reflect the centrality of intention in Catholic thought. As the Vatican "Declaration" notes, an omission as well as an action could be condemned as euthanasia.

No Catholic thinkers argue that life-sustaining treatment must be provided unless the patient is dying. Some, however, present the case of the imminently dying patient as the standard case (if not the only one) in which life-sustaining treatment appropriately may be forgone. In *The Gospel of Life*, Pope John Paul II distinguishes euthanasia from forgoing of aggressive or disproportionate treatment, but he presents legitimate forgoing only in cases corresponding to *goseis*: "In such situations, when death is clearly imminent and inevitable, one can in conscience 'refuse forms of treatment that would only secure a precarious and burdensome prolongation of life.'" One Catholic scholar reads this passage to imply that with respect to the distinction between ordinary and extraordinary treatment, "Pope John Paul II seems to limit the distinction's application to those who are close to death."[43] Limitation to this condition is especially common with regard to artificial nutrition and hydration. Like May et al., the Pennsylvania bishops write that nutrition and hydration might be extraordinary for "an imminently terminal patient," if the means would fail to restore health or improve the patient's condition. "However, the patient in the persistent vegetative state is not imminently terminal. . . . The feeding . . . serving a life-sustaining purpose. Therefore, it remains an ordinary means of sustaining life and should be continued."[44] For many conservative Catholic thinkers, although most medical treatments may be forgone in a variety of circumstances, it is difficult to justify forgoing artificial nutrition and hydration unless these means are therapeutically ineffective or merely prolong the dying of a patient in a *goseis* state.

Benefits and Burdens, Broadly Construed

A third set of approaches generally agrees with those discussed in the preceding section but takes a broader view of the benefits and burdens of treatment. In addition to concerns with burdens and questions regarding the obligatory nature of medical interventions, the claim is made that in some circumstances continuation of life may not benefit the patient. As expressed by David Kelly, "not all treatments which prolong biological life are humanly beneficial to the patient."[45] Although there is no sharp break between the approaches discussed in this section and those in the preceding section, those in this section tend to frame treatment decisions more clearly in terms of benefits and burdens and to understand these rubrics more expansively. Effective life-sustaining treatment might not be obligatory, even if the patient is not imminently dying and the treatment does not directly entail significant burdens, because the continuation of life would not be a significant benefit. Approaches focusing on benefits and burdens are dominant in the Roman Catholic tradition but also are found among some Jewish thinkers.

Conservative Jewish thinker Elliot Dorff advocates an approach that involves evaluating benefits and burdens for treatment decisions regarding terminally ill and permanently unconscious patients. Appealing to texts as well as experience, Dorff argues that "we should use the benefit to the patient as the primary criterion in determining a course of action rather than our ability to accomplish a limited medical goal (such as keeping one or more organs functioning)." A variety of medical treatments may be forgone on the basis of "our compassionate attention to the best interests of the patient" (as defined primarily by the patient, to the extent possible). Although a presumption supports provision of artificial nutrition and hydration, this presumption is rebuttable: These measures may be forgone for a terminally ill patient (at the request of the patient or surrogate) if they are considered not to serve the patient's best interests. Forgoing these interventions for a permanently unconscious patient is more difficult to justify. Decisions to forgo nutrition and hydration for these patients should not be made on the basis of the patient's quality of life, nor could they be made on the basis of risk (because death is certain if these means are forgone) or triage considerations (because feeding tubes are readily available). The argument could be made, however, that artificial nutrition and hydration represent medical means that are ineffective in curing permanently unconscious patients; when they do not serve the patient's best interests, they may be forgone.[46]

As I note above, evaluation of treatment in terms of benefits and burdens has provided the basic framework for decisions near the end of life in the Roman Catholic tradition. In the sixteenth century Vitoria judged that life-sustaining measures could be forgone if they offered little hope or entailed excessive personal or economic burdens. Similarly, Pope Pius XII ruled that only ordinary treatment is required, and individuals could reject means that impose a "grave burden for oneself or another." The 1980 Vatican "Declaration" authorized forgoing of extraordinary, or disproportionate, treatment. The traditional distinction between ordinary and extraordinary treatment, as summarized by Gerald Kelly, has been widely accepted by diverse Catholic thinkers as well as magisterial documents. The U.S. bishops' "Ethical and Religious Directives for Catholic Health Care Services" reflects this consensus: "A person has a moral obligation to use ordinary or proportionate means of preserving his or her life. . . . A person may forgo extraordinary or disproportionate means of preserving life. Disproportionate means are those that in the patient's judgment do not offer a reasonable hope of benefit or entail an excessive burden or impose excessive expense on the family or the community."[47]

Benefits and burdens generally have been construed fairly broadly, following the model of Gerald Kelly and his predecessors. Even the relatively conservative statement of May et al., which requires artificial nutrition and hydration for permanently unconscious patients, accepts an expansive view of burdens:

> Traditionally, a treatment has been judged useless or relatively useless if the benefits it provides to a person are nil (useless in a strict sense) or are insignificant in comparison to the burdens it imposes (useless in a wider sense). Traditionally, a treatment has been judged excessively burdensome when whatever benefits it offers are not worth pursuing for one or more of several reasons: It is too painful, too damaging to the patient's bodily self and functioning, too psychologically repugnant to the patient, too restrictive of the patient's liberty and preferred activities, too suppressive of the patient's mental life, or too expensive.[48]

For these writers, however, burdens involved in artificially feeding permanently unconscious patients are not significant; hence their view (noted above) that these measures must be provided.

Ashley and O'Rourke further expand the evaluation of burdens and benefits. They understand the key issue in treatment decisions to be the "proportion of benefits to burdens"; any form of care—not only medical treatment—may be forgone if it is disproportionately burdensome. Treatment may be forgone whenever it imposes a "grave burden" or fails to be "truly beneficial," even for patients who are not imminently dying. Burdens to be considered include not only those directly entailed by treatment but also "the burdens of total care." For permanently unconscious patients, burdens include "the indignity of existing in a state of persistent cognitive-affective deprivation [which] can be counted as a serious burden to the patient, even if the patient is unconscious," as well as burdens experienced by the family and caregivers.[49] A statement by Texas bishops emphasizes burdens experienced by others in judging that artificial nutrition and hydration could be forgone for permanently unconscious patients.[50]

The U.S. bishops' "Ethical and Religious Directives" states that "there should be a presumption in favor of providing nutrition and hydration to all patients, including patients who require medically assisted nutrition and hydration, as long as this is of sufficient benefit to outweigh the burdens involved to the patient." This document notes a consensus of bishops that these measures may be forgone in some cases in which they would be physiologically futile or if a patient is imminently dying but observes that there is no consensus regarding decisions for patients in a persistent vegetative state.[51] A statement on nutrition and hydration by the U.S. bishops' pro-life commission clearly reflects the common ground shared by Catholic authorities—and somewhat less clearly straddles the disputes they represent. Persons making judgments about nutrition and hydration may legitimately consider "physical risks and burden," "psychological burdens on the patient," and "economic and other burdens on caregivers." In judging psychological burdens, however, only "repugnance to the particular procedure" (not "repugnance to life itself") may be considered. Burdens on others must be judged with caution; it would be wrong to bring about the patient's death because of the patient's "imposing burdens on others." The bishops' only clear endorsement for forgoing of nutrition and hydration is for patients in "the final stage of a terminal condition"—corresponding to the *goseis* state—although they do not explicitly oppose forgoing of nutrition and hydration in all other conditions. They observe that "in the context of official church teaching, it is not yet clear to what extent we may assess the burden of a patient's total care rather than the burden of a particular treatment when we seek to refuse 'burdensome' life support." With regard to permanently unconscious patients they articulate a position that is similar to that expressed by Dorff, though with even greater caution:

> Decisions about these patients should be guided by a presumption in favor of medically assisted nutrition and hydration. A decision to discontinue such measures should be made in light of a careful assessment of the burdens and benefits of nutrition and hydration for the individual patient and his or her family and community. Such measures must not be withdrawn in order to cause death, but they may be withdrawn if they offer no reasonable hope of sustaining life or pose excessive risks or burdens.[52]

Diverse Catholic writers give prominence to burdens faced by others in making decisions about life-sustaining treatment. Explicit attention to burdens faced by the family or community has been noted in the bishops' "Ethical and Religious Directives," and by May et al. as well as Ashley and O'Rourke. Such burdens may be taken into account not only by the patient himself or herself but also by others who are experiencing burdens in caring for a patient without decisional capacity. With regard to resuscitation Pope Pius XII declares, "If it appears that the attempt at resuscitation constitutes in reality such a burden for the family that one cannot in all conscience impose it upon them, they can lawfully insist that the doctor should discontinue these attempts, and the doctor can lawfully comply." Ashley and O'Rourke state more generally, "If a patient can judge that some form of care is excessively burdensome, so can the patient's proxy when the patient becomes incompetent to make such a decision. Today one must also consider the burden to society."[53] For the Texas bishops, "examples of disproportionate burdens include excessive suffering for the patient; excessive expense for the family or the community; investment in medical technology and personnel disproportionate to the expected results; inequitable resource allocation."[54]

Jewish writers tend to be less willing to justify forgoing life-sustaining treatment for a patient because of burdens their care imposes on others. An exception is represented by Dorff, who justifies diverting resources from terminally ill patients to others on the grounds that these patients have a lower status than others in Jewish law.[55] Most Jewish thinkers, however, are reluctant to deprive one patient of resources needed to sustain life because of the needs of others.[56] This view also is reflected in the reluctance of Jewish thinkers to support rationing of health care resources, as discussed in chapter 7.

Pursuit of Life's Purpose and Quality of Life

Some Catholic thinkers have moved beyond even the foregoing relatively broad construal of benefits and burdens. They turn to a normative understanding of life's purpose as a basis for determining when sustaining life has value. Interventions that foster pursuit of life's purpose are obligatory; those that fail to serve or distract from life's purpose are optional, if not counterproductive. Writers who frame decisions this way may regard themselves as simply articulating the most reasonable specification of benefits and burdens, as discussed in the preceding section. For opponents, however, decisions to limit treatment on the basis of judgments that the patient's life objectively lacks sufficient value are more troubling than decisions that focus on the patient's own subjective experience of benefits and burdens.[57]

Richard McCormick presents the development of approaches that focus on life's purpose and the quality of life:

> Contemporary medicine . . . can keep almost anyone alive. This has tended gradually to shift the problem from the means to reverse the dying process to the quality of the life sustained and preserved. The questions, "Is this means too hazardous or difficult to use?" and "Does this measure only preserve the patient's dying?" while still useful and valid, now often become "Granted that we can easily save the life, what kind of life are we saving?" This is a quality-of-life judgment.[58]

McCormick appeals to the statement of Pope Pius XII that extraordinary means of preserving life are not required, in part because "a more strict obligation would be too burdensome for most men" but also because such an obligation "would render the attainment of the higher, more important good too difficult." For McCormick, the purpose of life is love of God—which is best expressed in relations with other humans—and love of neighbor. Accordingly, "the meaning, substance, and consummation of life are found in human relationships." Excessive efforts to sustain physical life distort values and distract from the pursuit of life's proper purpose.[59] Similarly, Kevin O'Rourke interprets Pius XII as "explicitly presenting the spiritual goal of life as the norm for judging whether a grave burden is present." Ordinary means to preserve life are "those means which are obligatory because they enable a person to strive for the spiritual purpose of life. 'Extraordinary' means would seem to be: those means which are optional because they are ineffective or a grave burden in helping a person strive for the spiritual purpose of life."[60] Writers offer various formulations of the purpose of life: "to know God, to love God, and to serve God by serving and loving our neighbor," "to strive for eternal life," drawing closer to God and returning God's love, "personal salvation and eternal happiness." Writers may also appeal generally to the "spiritual purpose of life," "life's goals and purposes," or "the humanly meaningful purposes of life."[61] However defined, the purpose of life becomes the basis for judging which treatments are appropriate and which are not. "A person may reject life-prolonging procedures if sustaining life does not help him or her strive for the purpose of life."[62]

For most writers who follow this approach, the purpose of life is not only used as a basis to judge particular interventions as supportive of or detracting from that purpose. One also may judge an individual's life as lacking any capacity to pursue life's purpose—in which case any intervention to sustain life would be extraordinary. Ashley and O'Rourke argue, "To prolong life, therefore, is of benefit only when it gives the person opportunity to continue to strive to achieve the spiritual purpose of life." When pursuit of life's purpose becomes impossible—as it does for permanently unconscious patients—any life-sustaining treatment, however simple or benign, would be extraordinary. "To pursue the spiritual purpose of life, one needs a minimal degree of cognitive-affective function. Therefore, if this function in an adult cannot be restored or if an infant will never develop this function, and if a fatal disease if **present, the adult** or infant may be allowed to die."[63]

Many writers who argue that no interventions need sustain the lives of persons who are incapable of pursuing life's purpose frame their arguments in terms of quality of life. These thinkers caution that quality-of-life judgments must be patient-centered rather than assessments of productivity or social utility. In part, quality-of-life judgments reflect the patient's experience of benefits and burdens (as discussed above). Attention to quality of life emphasizes that all of the benefits and burdens of the patient's life—not just those intrinsically connected to treatment modalities—must be considered. Some thinkers argue that Catholic tradition provides precedent for such judgments regarding the patient's life. Although traditional sources discuss the benefits and burdens of means, "often enough it is the kind of, the quality of the life thus saved (painful, poverty-stricken and deprived, away from home and friends, oppressive) that establishes the means as extraordinary. That type of life would be an excessive hardship for the individual."[64] Kevin Wildes argues that concerns regarding burdens "are not simply about the means or the quality of life during treatment, but also about the quality of life after treatment." If a patient could legitimately refuse an amputation (with anesthesia) because of "repugnance to living with a mutilated body," then a patient who already has experienced an amputation or other chronic infirmity should be able to refuse any life-sustaining treatment. The benefits and burdens of either decision are identical: additional life in a condition of amputation.[65]

"Quality of life" can refer not only to the patient's subjective sense of the benefits and burdens of existence but also to the patient's capacity to pursue the purpose of life. "The Roman Catholic tradition," David Kelly writes, "has recognized both the sanctity of life—life is indeed sacred—and the ethical import of at least some degree of quality of life—life need not be prolonged under all circumstances, that is, at some point a lack of the ability to carry out the humanly meaningful purposes of life, which some would call a lack of quality of life, means that life can be let go."[66] McCormick—a pioneer in developing the approach discussed in this section—includes in "quality of life" both the subjective experience of benefits and burdens and the capacity to pursue life's purpose. Life without potential for pursuing its purpose would not offer significant benefit to a patient. Overly aggressive treatment would impose the burden of distracting the patient from pursuing life's purpose and would leave the individual in a condition that "would distort and jeopardize his grasp on the overall meaning of life. Why? Because, it can be argued, human relationships—which are the very possibility of growth in love of God and neighbor—would be so threatened, strained, or submerged that they would no longer function as the heart and meaning of the individual's life as they should."[67]

Advocates of such quality of-life judgments acknowledge a need for caution in their application. An individual who is weakened but still able to pursue life's purpose to some extent must be accorded equal value with those enjoying more robust capabilities. "It is the pride of Judaeo-Christian tradition that the weak and defenseless, the powerless and unwanted, those whose grasp on the goods of life is most fragile—that is, those whose potential is real but reduced—are cherished and protected as our neighbor in greatest need." Even those without any capacity to pursue life's value remain human beings "of incalculable worth," though it may no longer make sense to prolong their biological life.[68] Some writers argue that although all life has ontic value—generating a *prima facie* duty to support its prolongation—when there is no capacity to pursue life's purpose, competing considerations may suggest that the limits to the actual duty of sustaining life have been reached.[69]

Some Catholic thinkers criticize arguments that a person's inability to pursue life's purpose, or a person's lack of quality of life, could provide a basis to forgo life-sustaining treatment. According to John Connery, traditional writers utilize not a quality of life norm but a "quality of treatment norm." Quality of life might be considered in judging the burdens and efficacy of treatment. However, to judge life itself in a given condition to be not worth living risks "euthanasia by omission." For Connery, the intent of Pius XII in the passage to which McCormick appeals is to explain why extraordinary means (understood in the sense of burdensome treatment) are not obligatory; when McCormick interprets Pius to suggest that there is no obligation to prolong life that lacks capacity, he goes "radically beyond anything the Pontiff had in mind." The duty to preserve life applies to all life and derives from the obligation to respect all life as a basic good.[70] Similarly, Barry criticizes the argument that there is no obligation to sustain the life of permanently unconscious patients: "It is also quite discriminatory because it implies that capacity for psychological relating is the ground for the possession of moral rights."[71]

The U.S. bishops' statement on nutrition and hydration articulates a position that leans toward the conservative side in this dispute. The statement endorses concern with quality of life, but in limited ways—closer to the appeals accepted by Connery than those of McCormick and Wildes. Patients should receive appropriate treatment to alleviate suffering and in that way improve their quality of life. Quality of life may be considered in the sense that patients may "refuse a treatment because it would itself create an impairment imposing new serious burdens or risks." Moreover, a patient with a disabling condition such as dementia may experience a treatment such as nutrition and hydration as "more frightening and burdensome" than would other patients. The document warns, however, against judgments that a life of limited quality need not be prolonged. "It is one thing to withhold a procedure because it would impose new disabilities on a patient, and quite another thing to say that patients who already have such disabilities should not have their lives preserved."[72] Although Ashley and O'Rourke generally agree with McCormick's position regarding the capacity to pursue life's goals, they avoid reference to the quality of life.[73]

Virtually all Jewish ethicists are hesitant to make judgments with regard to a patient's quality of life—or even to use this concept in bioethical deliberation. Even when concerns of the sort often associated with quality-of-life judgments are voiced by some Reform thinkers, explicit judgments about "quality of life" are studiously avoided. A document from the Reform movement expresses this position:

> It is clear that . . . we should do our best to enhance the quality of life and to use whatever means modern science has placed at our disposal for this purpose. We need not invoke "heroic" measures to prolong life, nor should we hesitate to alleviate pain, but we can also not utilize a "low quality" of life as an excuse for hastening death.[74]

Many Jewish thinkers, including some Orthodox authorities, would be sympathetic to Pius XII's consideration to forgo treatment that "would be too burdensome for most" people. Few would be as ready to forgo life-sustaining treatment in the name of a "higher, more important good" or as concerned that preserving life and health might interfere with a "more serious duty."

Conclusion

In this chapter I note extensive similarities between Jewish and Roman Catholic approaches to treatment decisions near the end of life. Writers in the two traditions appeal to similar values and concerns in addressing this topic. The traditions share a commitment to the value of life and the responsibility to provide healing to persons in need, as well as an obligation for patients to accept appropriate medical treatment. Both traditions agree that patients have some range of autonomous choice but that, at least as a moral matter, this range is constrained by objective moral limits. Medical interventions may be refused in some cases, particularly when these measures are excessively burdensome or lacking benefit. Nevertheless, there is a concern in both communities that not all refusals of life-sustaining treatment are morally licit.

Within this broad consensus there are a variety of more particular views. Jewish and Catholic positions on these issues represent overlapping spectra, with the Jewish spectrum extending somewhat to the right—expressing greater reluctance to forgo medical interventions. At one extreme, some Orthodox Jewish authorities require continuation of life-sustaining treatment in virtually all circumstances. Many Jewish and some Catholic thinkers agree that life represents an intrinsic benefit but would allow forgoing of treatment, especially for a dying patient, when treatment would be therapeutically ineffective or merely would prolong the dying process. The view of thinkers such as Robert Barry and William E. May that artificial nutrition and hydration must be provided unless they are ineffective or intrinsically burdensome, at the right end of the Catholic spectrum, would be closer to the center of the Jewish range. Most Catholic and some Jewish writers would evaluate treatment decisions in terms of benefits and burdens, broadly construed, authorizing forgoing of treatment in a wider range of cases. Finally, some Catholic thinkers appeal to the quality of life and the patient's ability to pursue life's goals, judging any intervention pointless if it fails to support such a pursuit.

A variety of factors may help to account for the differences observed between Jewish and Catholic writers. For Jews across a spectrum of beliefs, even more than for Catholic thinkers, saving and preserving life is a cardinal precept, superseding virtually all duties. Jewish theologians probably are affected by a history marked by centuries of discrimination and mistreatment, including the Holocaust. Because the Nazis used phrases such as "life not worthy of life," Jewish thinkers are reluctant even to speak of quality-of-life judgments (even with the care and caution expressed by Catholic theologians who use these terms). Following mass killings of Jews and threats to physical survival, these theologians may lean more heavily to the side of life in maintaining life-sustaining treatment.

Divergences in general tendencies also may reflect more general differences in doctrine or central narratives. Some people claim that Judaism is a "this-worldly" religion and Christianity "other-worldly." Although this claim is oversimplified, it does reflect an element of truth. For many Catholic theologians, the central narrative of Jesus's death and resurrection has relativized the life of this world. Life in this world clearly is subordinated to spiritual development and life eternal. Although Jewish views on this subject are complex and varied, few Jewish theologians would put things quite that way. A typical Jewish understanding is that this world and life eternal represent two goods that are each basic and incommensurable, neither serving only instrumentally for the other.[75] At least at the margins, such an understanding of the value of this-worldly life would tend to support greater emphasis on preserving life.

Finally, although there are elements that might be seen as teleological and deontological in each tradition, Jewish theologians tend to give teleological analysis a less decisive role in ethical deliberations than do Catholic theologians. For many diverse Catholic thinkers, the patterns of nature and the appropriate ends of the human person can be known with a significant degree of precision and confidence. Ethical judgments tend to derive from these understandings of humans and the world. Jewish thinkers tend to be more modest in claims regarding knowledge of patterns and purposes and to judge that ethical responsibilities may be known with greater precision and confidence.[76] Accordingly, Catholic writers more commonly articulate a normative model of human life and purposes and use this model as a basis for practical decisions that some life-sustaining interventions are inappropriate. Jewish writers more commonly understand the obligation to preserve life as decisive in practice.

I compare Jewish and Catholic approaches more fully in the conclusion to this book. In chapter 5 I examine the bioethics issue that reflects the greatest divergence between these traditions, with Catholic writers tending toward the more conservative stance: abortion.

Notes

1. Gerald Kelly, *Medico-Moral Problems* (St. Louis: Catholic Health Association, 1958), 132.

2. See Daniel A. Cronin, "Concerning Human Life," in *Concerning Human Life*, ed. Russell E. Smith (Braintree, Mass.: Pope John XXIII Medical-Moral Research and Education Center, 1989); Robert Barry, "Feeding the Comatose and the Common Good in the Catholic Tradition," *Thomist* 53 (1989): 1–30; Kevin O'Rourke, "Evolution of Church Teaching on Prolonging Life," *Health Progress* 69, no. 1 (1988): 28–35; Richard A. McCormick, "To Save or Let Die: The Dilemma of Modern Medicine," in *How Brave a New World?* (Washington, D.C.: Georgetown University Press, 1981), 345–46; John R. Connery, "Quality of Life," *Linacre Quarterly* 53 (1986): 26–33.

3. For example, the Vatican's 1980 "Declaration on Euthanasia" condemns euthanasia—defined as "an action *or an omission* which of itself or by intention causes death, in order that all suffering may in this way be eliminated" (Congregation for the Doctrine of the Faith, *Origins* 10 [1980]: 155; emphasis added). Avram Israel Reisner of the Jewish Conservative movement states that "the permission to seek hospice care is a life-affirming permission. One may not choose hospice care so as to die more quickly, but rather, only in order to live one's remaining days in the best way possible"; see "Care for the Terminally Ill: Halakhic Concepts and Values," in *Life and Death Responsibilities in Jewish Biomedical Ethics*, ed. Aaron L. Mackler (New York: Jewish Theological Seminary of America, Finkelstein Institute, 2000), 252.

4. *Relectiones Theologiae* and *Comentarios a la Seconda Secundae de Santo Tomas*, in Cronin, "Concerning Human Life," 34–38; see also O'Rourke, "Evolution of Church Teaching on Prolonging Life," 29; Barry, "Feeding the Comatose," 5–9. Although the use of medicine is not required,

it generally is commendable. "They are not to be condemned of mortal sin who have universally declared an abstinence from drugs, although this is not laudable because God created medicine because of its need" (*Relectiones*, in Cronin, "Concerning Human Life," 35).

5. *De Justitia et Jure*, Disp. 10, section 1, in Cronin, "Concerning Human Life," 47–55; see also Barry, "Feeding the Comatose," 9–11. As noted below, later Catholic tradition provides greater latitude for a patient to reject amputation, even with anesthesia.

6. Kelly, *Medico-Moral Problems* 129 (emphasis in original).

7. Pope Pius XII, "The Prolongation of Life," *The Pope Speaks* 4 (1958): 395–96.

8. Congregation for the Doctrine of the Faith, "Declaration on Euthanasia" 155–56.

9. *Shulḥan Arukh*, *Yoreh Deah* 336:1; Talmud, *Yoma* 83a–85a. The Mishnah states, "If debris fall on someone, and it is doubtful whether or not he is there, or whether he is alive or dead . . . one should open the heap of debris for his sake [even on the Sabbath]. If one finds him alive one should remove the debris, and if he be dead one should leave him [until after the Sabbath]." The Talmud queries, "'If one finds him alive one should remove the debris?'—but that is self-evident [and does not need to be stated]. No, the statement is necessary, to show that even for the life of the hour [i.e., with only a short while to live], we dig on the Sabbath."

10. The cases of a person covered by rubble and a person being burned to death are different. It is possible that de Lugo would support excavating a person to prolong life by a few hours, and the Talmud might not require prolonging the process of being burned, as may be reflected in the case of Rabbi Ḥanina discussed below. Nonetheless, de Lugo provides a precedent influencing Catholic thinkers to doubt the value of briefly prolonging life, and the Talmud offers a precedent influencing Jewish thinkers to affirm that value.

11. *Shulḥan Arukh*, *Yoreh Deah* 339. This text is taken originally from the sixth-century tractate *Semaḥot*. As I note subsequently, the precise referent of the term *goseis* is a matter of dispute.

12. *Mapah* to *Shulḥan Arukh*, *Yoreh De'ah* 339. The original source of this passage—the twelfth-century *Sefer Ḥasidim*—as well as Isserles's commentary to another code state that not only is one not obligated to prolong the dying process but that one should not "cause a person not to die quickly when he is a *goseis*" (*Darkhei Moshe* to *Tur*, *Yoreh De'ah* 339; *Sefer Ḥasidim*, n. 723). *Sefer Ḥasidim* similarly states (n. 234), "'A time to die': Why does Kohelet (Ecclesiastes) say this? If a man is a *goseis*, when the man's soul is departing, one does not shout so that the soul would return, for he could only live a few days, and during that time he would suffer."

13. B. *Avodah Zarah* 18a.

14. See Louis E. Newman, "Woodchoppers and Respirators: The Problem of Interpretation in Contemporary Jewish Ethics," in *Contemporary Jewish Ethics and Morality*, ed. Elliot N. Dorff and Louis E. Newman (New York: Oxford University Press, 1995), 141–49; Basil F. Herring, *Jewish Ethics and Halakhah for Our Time* (New York: Ktav and Yeshiva University Press, 1984), 79–86; Avraham Steinberg, *Encyclopedia of Jewish Medical Ethics*, vol. 4 (Jerusalem: Schlesinger Institute, 1988–98), s.v. "Terminally Ill" [*Noteh Lamut*], 365–75; J. David Bleich, "The Obligation to Heal in the Judaic Tradition: A Comparative Analysis," in *Jewish Bioethics*, ed. Fred Rosner and J. David Bleich (New York: Sanhedrin, 1979), 33–35; Reisner, "Care for the Terminally Ill," 245–47.

15. Immanuel Jakobovits, *Jewish Medical Ethics*, rev. ed. (New York: Bloch, 1975), 276 (emphasis in original); Bleich, "Obligation to Heal," 29, 17–20. As I note, Jakobovits's own views of treatment decisions are not as vitalist as this quote might suggest.

16. Bleich, "Obligation to Heal," 33–35; Eliezer Yehudah Waldenberg, *Tzitz Eliezer*, 2d ed. (Jerusalem, Israel: n.p., 1985), vol. 5, *Ramat Rahel*, nn. 28–29; vol. 13, n. 89.

17. Steinberg, *Encyclopedia of Jewish Medical Ethics*, vol. 4, 368–72; Baruch A. Brody, "A Historical Introduction to Jewish Casuistry on Suicide and Euthanasia," in *Suicide and Euthanasia: Historical and Contemporary Themes*, ed. Baruch A. Brody (Dordrecht, Netherlands: Kluwer, 1989), 66; Reisner, "Care for the Terminally Ill," 246–47.

18. Shlomo Zalman Auerbach, *Minhat Shlomo* (Jerusalem: Sha'arei Ziv Institute, 5746 [1985/6]), n. 91:24, p. 558; Hayyim David Halevi, "Disconnecting a Patient with no Prospect of Survival from a Respirator," *Tehumin* 2 (5741 [1980/81]): 303–5. See also Baruch A. Brody, "Jewish Reflections on Life and Death Decision Making," in *Jewish and Catholic Bioethics: An Ecumenical Dialogue*, ed. Edmund D. Pellegrino and Alan I. Faden (Washington, D.C.: Georgetown University Press, 1999), 19.

19. Steinberg, *Encyclopedia of Jewish Medical Ethics*, vol. 4, 367–70; Herring, *Jewish Ethics and Halakhah for Our Time*, 85–87. Steinberg (369–70) cites one authority who argues that one may not hasten death when the soul wants to remain but may remove hindrances when the soul wishes to depart; Steinberg observes that from a medical perspective this distinction is impossible to apply in practice. Moshe D. Tendler and Fred Rosner cite the ruling of Solomon Eger that "it is forbidden to hinder the departure of the soul by the use of medicines." They conclude, "To prolong life is a *mitsva*, to prolong dying is not"; Moshe D. Tendler and Fred Rosner, "Quality and Sanctity of Life in the Talmud and the Midrash," *Tradition* 28, no. 1 (1993): 20, 26.

20. David M. Feldman, *Health and Medicine in the Jewish Tradition* (New York: Crossroad, 1986), 95.

21. *A Time to Prepare*, ed. Richard F. Address (Philadelphia: Union of American Hebrew Congregations, n.d.), 36, quoting Bernard Zlotowitz.

22. Immanuel Jacobovits, "Whether It Is Permitted to Hasten the Death of a Terminally Ill Patient Who Is Suffering," *Hapardes* 31, no. 3 (1956): 18–19. Jakobovits rules that forgoing insulin would be acceptable even if the patient, while terminally ill, has not yet reached the stage of *goseis*.

23. Moshe Feinstein, *Iggerot Moshe*, vol. 7 (Bnei Berak, Israel: Ohel Yosef, 1985), Ḥoshen Mishpat 2, n. 74, pp. 311–12. Feinstein holds, however, that if the patient is not suffering life-sustaining treatment should be provided.

24. Gedaliah Aharon Rabinowitz and Mordecai Koenigsberg, "The Definition of Death and Determination of Its Time according to Halakhah," *Hadarom* no. 32 (1970): 75.

25. Central Conference of American Rabbis, "On the Treatment of the Terminally Ill," in *Teshuvot for the Nineties: Reform Judaism's Answers for Today's Dilemmas* (New York: Central Conference of American Rabbis, 1997), 348 (emphasis in original).

26. Auerbach, *Minḥat Shlomo* 91:24, and Steinberg, *Encyclopedia of Jewish Medical Ethics,* vol. 4, 403.

27. Israel Ministry of Health, Report of the Steinberg Commission on the Care of the Terminally Ill Patient, 2002, Proposed Legislation, sections 2, 6, 10–13 (available at www.health.gov.il/pages/default.asp?PageId=632&parentId=10&catId=6&maincat=1). Artificial nutrition and hydration are among the routine measures to be continued, unless specifically refused by a competent patient despite efforts at persuasion (section 10).

28. Reisner, "Care for the Terminally Ill: Practical Applications," in *Life and Death Responsibilities in Jewish Biomedical Ethics*, ed. Aaron L. Mackler (New York: Jewish Theological Seminary of America, Finkelstein Institute, 2000), 265–69; idem, "Care for the Terminally Ill: Halakhic Values," 243. See also the options authorized by Reisner in the Conservative "Jewish Medical Directives for Health Care," *Life and Death Responsibilities*, 374–81.

29. These writers, however, might accord less scope than does Reisner for forgoing treatment on the basis of uncertainty and the intrinsic burdens of treatment.

30. *Appointment of a Health Care Agent/Advance Directive* (New York: Rabbinical Council of America, n.d.); Tendler and Rosner, "Quality and Sanctity of Life," 26.

31. Steinberg, *Encyclopedia of Jewish Medical Ethics,* vol. 4, 405–6; Rabbinical Council of America, *Appointment of a Health Care*

Agent/Advance Directive. For the Steinberg Commission, artificial nutrition and hydration represent routine treatment that must be provided in virtually all cases, unless refused by a competent patient despite attempts to persuade him or her to accept these interventions, or when an advance directive provides clear evidence of refusal for a patient lacking capacity who is in the final two weeks of life and is suffering (sections 10, 13).

32. Reisner, "Care for the Terminally Ill: Practical Applications," 266–67.

33. Steinberg, *Encyclopedia of Jewish Medical Ethics*, vol. 4, 405–6.

34. Central Conference of American Rabbis, "On the Treatment of the Terminally Ill," 354–55. This deference to individual conscience accords with the general approach of Reform Judaism, as discussed in chapter 2.

35. Steinberg, *Encyclopedia of Jewish Medical Ethics*, vol. 4, 413–14; Rabbinical Council of America, *Appointment of a Health Care Agent/Advance Directive.*

36. Reisner, "Care for the Terminally Ill: Practical Applications," 272–73. See also the options authorized by Reisner in the Conservative "Jewish Medical Directives for Health Care" in Mackler, *Life and Death Responsibilities*, 381–82.

37. Rabinowitz and Koenigsberg, "Definition of Death and Determination of Its Time," 75.

38. Steinberg, *Encyclopedia of Jewish Medical Ethics*, vol. 4, 406–7.

39. Steinberg Commission, Report on the Care of the Terminally Ill Patient, sections 12–13.

40. Halevi, "Disconnecting a Patient with No Prospect of Survival," 304–5.

41. Feldman, *Health and Medicine in the Jewish Tradition*, 95. Conservative writer Elliot Dorff argues that "it is easier to justify withdrawing a treatment that has proven not beneficial than not to try a possibly beneficial therapy at all;" see "End-Stage Medical Care: Practical Applications," in Mackler, *Life and Death Responsibilities*, 339–40.

42. William E. May et al., "Feeding and Hydrating the Permanently Unconscious and Other Vulnerable Persons," *Issues in Law and Medicine* 3, no. 3 (1987): 203–17 (emphasis in original). Among the signatories to this statement is Jewish thinker David Novak. See also Barry, "Feeding the Comatose," 17: "To withhold these forms of care would be morally equivalent to killing by omission." Additional authors are noted in Lisa Sowle Cahill, "Notes on Moral Theology: Bioethical Decisions to End Life," *Theological Studies* 52 (1991): 110–14.

43. John Paul II, *Evangelium Vitae: The Gospel of Life* (Washington, D.C.: United States Catholic Conference, 1995), n. 65, p. 117, citing

"Declaration on Euthanasia"; Kevin W. Wildes, "Ordinary and Extraordinary Means and the Quality of Life," *Theological Studies* 57 (1996): 509. Benedict M. Ashley and Kevin D. O'Rourke acknowledge that the pope discusses the forgoing of treatment only in cases of imminent death but argue that because he cites the "Declaration on Euthanasia" he would agree with the broader scope of forgoing extraordinary treatment in that document. He simply chooses "to illustrate the criterion of benefit versus burden with the most obvious and uncontroverted case" (Benedict M. Ashley and Kevin D. O'Rourke, *Health Care Ethics: A Theological Analysis*, 4th ed. [Washington, D.C.: Georgetown University Press, 1997], 422).

44. Bishops of Pennsylvania, "Nutrition and Hydration: Moral Considerations," *Origins* 21 (1992): 548. See similarly New Jersey Catholic Conference, "Providing Food and Fluids to Severely Brain Damaged Patients," *Origins* 16 (1987): 582–84. As I discuss, other groups of bishops present differing views on forgoing artificial nutrition and hydration from a patient in a persistent vegetative state.

45. David F. Kelly, *Critical Care Ethics: Treatment Decisions in American Hospitals* (Kansas City, Mo.: Sheed and Ward, 1991), 1.

46. Dorff, "End-Stage Medical Care: Halakhic Concepts and Values," in *Life and Death Responsibilities*, 311–15; "End-Stage Medical Care: Practical Applications," 344, 348–54. See also the options authorized by Dorff in the Conservative "Jewish Medical Directives for Health Care" in Mackler, *Life and Death Responsibilities*, 374–81. Dorff writes, "nutrition and hydration . . . are needed by everyone. Therefore, the burden of proof shifts: One needs to justify the *use* of medications, but one needs to justify the *failure* to provide nutrition and hydration" ("End-Stage Medical Care: Practical Applications," 349; emphasis in original).

47. National Conference of Catholic Bishops, "Ethical and Religious Directives for Catholic Health Care Services," *Origins* 24 (1994), nn. 56–57, p. 459.

48. May et al., "Feeding and Hydrating the Permanently Unconscious and Other Vulnerable Persons," 208.

49. Ashley and O'Rourke, *Health Care Ethics*, 421–23.

50. Texas Bishops, "On Withholding Artificial Nutrition and Hydration," *Origins* 20 (1990): 54. Patients in a persistent vegetative state "are stricken with a lethal pathology which, without artificial nutrition and hydration, will lead to death. . . . The morally appropriate forgoing or withdrawing of artificial nutrition and hydration from a permanently unconscious person is not abandoning that person. Rather, it is accepting the fact that the person has come to the end of his or her pilgrimage and should not be impeded from taking the final step." This statement was issued by sixteen of eighteen

Texas bishops. See the similar Oregon and Washington Bishops', "Living and Dying Well," *Origins* 21 (1991): 350. For a review of bishops' statements on this issue, see James F. Keenan and Myles Sheehan, "Life Supports: Sorting Bishops' Views," *Church* (winter 1992), 10–17.

51. U.S. Bishops, "Ethical and Religious Directives," n. 58 and Introduction to part 5, pp. 458–59.

52. National Conference of Catholic Bishops Committee for Pro-Life Activities, "Nutrition and Hydration: Moral and Pastoral Reflections," *Origins* 21 (1992): 706–10.

53. Pope Pius XII, "The Prolongation of Life," 397; Ashley and O'Rourke, *Health Care Ethics*, 424. See also Jean deBlois and Kevin D. O'Rourke, "Issues at the End of Life," *Health Progress* 76, no. 6 (1995): 25.

54. Texas Bishops, "On Withholding Artificial Nutrition and Hydration," 54.

55. Dorff, "End-Stage Medical Care: Practical Applications," 340–44. Baruch Brody, "Jewish Reflections," 22–23, argues that burdens on society may be taken into account in determining the extent of society's responsibility to provide needed health care.

56. Shimon Glick claims, "The only concern of the *halakhah* is the welfare of the patient under discussion. It is clear when one reads much of the general literature on the subject that all too often it is the interests of the family, the staff, and/or the society that may influence the decision, usually in a direction of terminating the patient's life. These considerations are totally unacceptable by our tradition" ("The Jewish Approach to Living and Dying," in *Jewish and Catholic Bioethics*, 51). See also the statement of May et al., "Feeding and Hydrating the Permanently Unconscious," 211: "It is possible to imagine situations in which a society might reasonably consider it too burdensome to continue to care for its helpless members. . . . However, our society is by no means in such straitened circumstances—in the aftermath of nuclear destruction we may face such a situation, but we are surely not facing one now."

57. Secular philosopher John Arras has noted the potential divergence between criteria that are based on the patient's experience of benefits and burdens and those based on the capacity to pursue life's purpose. Arras considers the case of a profoundly retarded, blind, and deaf newborn who is not experiencing pain or other suffering but is merely "subsisting on the back ward." Arras argues that for this child, continued existence likely would represent a marginal benefit (hence, continued treatment would be supported by the standard described in the preceding section). Because of the infant's radical lack of human capabilities, however, continued life and therefore treatment would be valueless. Arras cites Richard McCormick's approach; he

agrees with McCormick that life-sustaining treatment would be inappropriate for persons radically lacking human capacities, but Arras writes that "McCormick confuses his standard based on lack of basic human capacities with the best-interest standard"; John D. Arras, "Toward an Ethic of Ambiguity," *Hastings Center Report* 14, no. 2 (1984): 31–33.

58. McCormick, "To Save or Let Die," 344–45.

59. Ibid., 345–46.

60. O'Rourke, "Evolution of Church Teaching on Prolonging Life," 32. Likewise, after quoting Pope Pius XII's statement, Ashley and O'Rourke, *Health Care Ethics*, 426, continue, "In other words, the means to prolong life may be withheld or withdrawn if these means do not help a person strive for the spiritual purpose of life, or if they impose a grave burden on the person or the person's caregivers in regard to striving for that purpose. This places the ethical question squarely in the context of the traditional Christian view that all our free decisions must be measured by our ultimate goal, eternal life with God."

61. deBlois and O'Rourke, "Issues at the End of Life," 24; O'Rourke, "Evolution of Church Teaching on Prolonging Life," 28–29; Wildes, "Ordinary and Extraordinary Means," 502; Ashley and O'Rourke, *Health Care Ethics*, 426; James J. Walter, "The Meaning and Validity of Quality of Life Judgments in Contemporary Roman Catholic Medical Ethics," *Louvain Studies* 13 (1988): 201; David Kelly, *Critical Care Ethics*, 5.

62. deBlois and O'Rourke, "Issues at the End of Life," 24.

63. Ashley and O'Rourke, *Health Care Ethics*, 426; O'Rourke, "Evolution of Church Teaching on Prolonging Life," 33. See similarly deBlois and O'Rourke, 27: "Prolonging the life of persons in PVS does not seem to enhance their ability to strive for the purpose and goods of life."

64. McCormick, "To Save or Let Die," 347. Similarly Cahill, "Notes on Moral Theology," 114: "If a particular means can prolong life but is still refused, then implicitly the life permitted to end has been judged in some sense not worth living."

65. Wildes, "Ordinary and Extraordinary Means," 505. "The assessment of a burdensome nature of a treatment is a quality-of-life judgment. Is the treatment itself a burden to the patient, or does the treatment leave the patient in a condition that the patient finds repugnant? Since there is no absolute standard by which to make these judgments, they will be relative to the patient's perception of his or her own life"; Wildes, "Ordinary and Extraordinary Means," 507.

66. David F. Kelly, *Critical Care Ethics*, 5. James Walter focuses on this aspect of quality of life, downplaying the aspect of subjective experience. The "quality" of concern is not so much an attribute of life but "the quality of the

relationship which exists between the medical condition of the patient, on the one hand, and the patient's ability to pursue life's goals and purposes (purposefulness) understood as the values that transcend physical life, on the other" (Walter, "Meaning and Validity of Quality of Life Judgments," 201). See Cahill, "Notes on Moral Theology," 116–18, who observes that Walter (and Thomas Shannon) seek to avoid some of the criticisms made against evaluating life in terms of quality (see below), but articulate a position fundamentally the same as that of McCormick.

67. McCormick, "To Save or Let Die," 347.

68. Ibid., 351, 350.

69. Walter, "Meaning and Validity of Quality of Life Judgments," 206; Cahill, "Notes on Moral Theology," 118.

70. Connery, "Quality of Life," 27, 30–32. Connery acknowledges that "there is a limit to the obligation to preserve life," but denies "that this limit is based on quality-of-life itself" (31).

71. Barry, "Feeding the Comatose," 14.

72. Pro-Life Committee, "Nutrition and Hydration" 709.

73. The only reference to "quality of life" in their index is to arguments by May and Grisez against the use of this term (Ashley and O'Rourke, *Health Care Ethics,* 422). The extent to which Ashley and O'Rourke's avoidance of this term reflects their concerns about possible abuse of the term and the extent to which it simply reflects deference to magisterial sensitivities are unclear.

74. Walter Jacob, ed., *Contemporary Reform Responsa* (New York: Central Conference of American Rabbis, 1987), 140. The passage continues, "We can not generalize about the 'quality of life' but must treat each case we face individually. All life is wonderful and mysterious. The human situation, the family setting and other factors must be carefully analyzed before a sympathetic decision can be reached."

75. See discussion in the Introduction and in the Conclusion.

76. Although this theme is not universal, it can be found in sources ranging from the book of Exodus to Emmanuel Levinas. See discussion in the Conclusion to this book.

Chapter 5

Abortion

AMONG THE ISSUES CONSIDERED IN THIS BOOK, ABORTION presents the greatest divergence between Roman Catholic and Jewish approaches. This divergence is especially dramatic at the theoretical level, with regard to the status of the fetus or unborn child. Catholic writers tend to regard the fetus as a person, with rights essentially equal to that of the mother and others, throughout at least most of pregnancy. Official church teaching, and many theologians, assert that the unborn child must be respected as a person from the time of conception; the overwhelming majority of writers would accord this status no later than the third week of gestation. Jewish thinkers hold that the fetus does not fully acquire the status of a person until birth. Some would grant the fetus a status almost equivalent to that of the pregnant woman; virtually all would acknowledge significant value to the fetus as representing potential life and the miraculous creation of God. The gap between the traditions persists but narrows somewhat on the practical issue of the acceptability of abortion; Jewish thinkers agree that abortion generally is wrong and justifiable only for significant reasons; some Catholic thinkers accept abortion for the most serious reasons, such as saving the mother's life.

In this chapter I survey briefly the historical development of discussion of this topic in each tradition. I then examine contemporary views, first regarding the status of the fetus or unborn child and then the acceptability of abortion in various circumstances. I also devote attention to the call of writers in each tradition to respond to broader issues raised by this topic, including the need to address causes of abortion. I conclude the chapter by summarizing points of agreement and disagreement between the traditions.

Historical Development

Both Judaism and Roman Catholicism have roots in the Hebrew Bible (also known as the Tanakh or Old Testament). Although the Hebrew Bible does not directly discuss the issue of abortion, it provides values and concepts that help to shape deliberation in each tradition. As I note in the introduction to this book, the Hebrew Bible reflects values of human life, compassion, healing, and procreation. One precedent that has been influential in the Jewish tradition is provided in the book of Exodus (21:22–23). "When men fight, and one of them pushes a pregnant woman and a miscarriage results, but no other damage ensues, the one responsible shall be fined according as the woman's husband may exact from him, the payment to be based on reckoning. But if other damage ensues, the penalty shall be life for life. . . ."[1] A significant variation is found in the Septuagint—the ancient Greek translation that became influential for Christianity but not for rabbinic Judaism: "If two men strive and smite a woman, and her child is imperfectly formed, he shall be forced to pay a penalty. . . . But if he be perfectly formed, he shall give life for life. . . ."[2] The Hebrew Bible also contains passages reflecting God's relationship with individuals before birth. Thus, Jeremiah is addressed by God: "Before I created you in the womb, I selected you; before you were born, I consecrated you" (Jeremiah 1:5).

Catholic Views

The New Testament continued the Hebrew Bible's commitments to the value of human life and God's concern for the weak. The significance of the unborn child is highlighted in the gospel infancy narratives. According to Luke (1:41, 44), the child within Elizabeth's womb (John the Baptist) leaped with joy at the greeting of Mary, with Jesus in her womb. The New Testament does not explicitly mention abortion, however.[3] An early explicit condemnation of abortion may be found in the first-century *Didache*: "You shall not kill. You shall not commit adultery. You shall not corrupt boys. You shall not fornicate. You shall not steal. You shall not make magic. You shall not practice medicine (*pharmakeia*). You shall not slay the child by abortions (*phthora*). You shall not kill what is generated. You shall not desire your neighbor's wife." Abortion was condemned as destroying what God had made.[4] Church fathers such as Augustine and Jerome condemned all abortions. For these authorities, abortion would represent homicide only after the formation of the fetus, some time after conception. Earlier abortion would be condemned as contraception, which was absolutely prohibited and could be considered equivalent to homicide.[5]

The medieval church consistently condemned all abortions. Generally, abortion was considered homicide only after the formation of the body and ensoulment—which was commonly understood to occur about the fortieth day after conception.[6] The first influential statement explicitly permitting abortion in some circumstances (rather than merely mitigating its penalty) appears to have been offered by John of Naples in the fourteenth century, as reported by Antoninus of Florence (fifteenth century). A physician generally should not give a pregnant woman medicine to cause abortion, even when necessary to save her life; when "one cannot help one without hurting the other, it is more appropriate to help neither." If the fetus is not yet animated or ensouled, however, the doctor "ought to give such medicine" because "although he impedes the ensoulment of a future fetus, he will not be the cause of the death of any man."[7] This permission was accepted by some authorities and rejected by others. Thomas Sanchez (sixteenth century) explicitly supports the view of John of Naples, arguing that the killing of an unanimated fetus would not constitute homicide and that in certain cases the fetus could be considered a "quasi-aggressor." Francis Torreblanca (seventeenth century) was unusual in extending permission for abortion to preserve the mother's reputation. Antonius de Corduba (sixteenth century) ruled that a medicine that would be therapeutic for the mother but would indirectly kill the fetus should be given; a medicine that would principally and directly kill the fetus, however, would be prohibited. This distinction between direct and indirect killing of the fetus became widely accepted.[8]

Beginning in the seventeenth century, the consensus on delayed ensoulment increasingly was challenged. Thomas Fienus argued that the fetus received a soul about the third day after conception. In 1621 Paolo Zacchia argued that the rational soul must be "infused in the first moment of conception." He accepted the lesser penalty of canon law for abortions before the fortieth day, however, believing that these early abortions entail a somewhat lesser injury than do later abortions.[9] In 1679 the Holy Office under Pope Innocent XI condemned several propositions, including two related to abortion:

34. It is lawful to procure abortion before ensoulment of the fetus lest a girl, detected as pregnant, be killed or defamed.
35. It seems probable that the fetus (as long as it is in the uterus) lacks a rational soul and begins first to have one when it is born; and consequently it must be said that no abortion is a homicide.[10]

Some authorities continued to accept abortion to save the mother from medical threat intrinsically imposed by pregnancy, which was not included in the condemned propositions, although it increasingly was rejected.

In the nineteenth century, Augustine Lehmkuhl accepted abortion of an animated fetus to save the mother's life as a probable (defensible) view because removing the fetus from the womb is not necessarily a direct killing. The fetus may be presumed to renounce being in the mother's womb, so abortion need not be regarded as killing—just as an individual may yield a plank to a friend following a shipwreck without his action being regarded as suicide. Lehmkuhl would not allow a direct attack on the fetus, such as a craniotomy or embryotomy. Such procedures were defended by a few thinkers, including Pietro Avanzini. Daniel Viscosi argued that the fetus could be considered a material aggressor; furthermore, the fetus would not suffer significant harm from such procedures in cases in which the fetus would die in any eventuality. Viscosi also argued that the killing of the fetus, even when physically direct in causation, could be considered indirect on the basis of the agent's intention. John Connery presents Viscosi's argument: "What is directly willed is saving the life of the mother. The surgeon does not want the death of the fetus. He does what he does only because he wants to save the mother." Also arguing for the acceptability of craniotomy was Joseph Pennacchi, who cites the passage from Exodus noted above to argue that the absolute prohibition of killing does not apply to the fetus.[11] Other thinkers argued against these claims. In 1884–95, the Vatican Holy Office issued a series of rulings that effectively prohibited all abortions, resolving for the magisterium the debate about abortion to save the mother's life. The debate regarding the status of the early fetus also was resolved by the magisterium in this period. In 1869 Pope Pius IX extended the penalty of excommunication for abortion from that of the "ensouled fetus" to all abortions.[12] In 1930 Pope Pius XI articulated the prohibition of any therapeutic abortion in his encyclical, *Casti Connubii*:

> As to the "medical and therapeutic indication" to which, using their own words, We have made reference, Venerable Brethren, however much we may pity the mother whose health and even life is gravely imperiled in the performance of the duty allotted to her by nature, nevertheless what could ever be a sufficient reason for excusing in any way the direct murder of the innocent? This is precisely what we are dealing with here.[13]

Abortion was later condemned by papal pronouncements, as well as by the Second Vatican Council. "Life must be protected with the utmost care from the moment of conception: abortion and infanticide are abominable crimes."[14]

Jewish Views

A central text in Jewish deliberations about abortion is found in the Mishnah, compiled around 200 C.E.:

> If a woman is having [life-threatening] difficulty giving birth, one dismembers the fetus within her and brings it forth limb by limb, because her life comes before its life. Once the greater part has emerged, one may not touch it, for one may not set aside one life (*nefesh*) to save another.[15]

All Jewish authorities agree that the fetus has a lesser status than that of the woman, although there is debate about whether this status is nearly equivalent to hers or significantly lower, which would provide greater scope for permissible abortions. All Jewish authorities agree that abortion is permitted to save the woman's life, although the permissibility of abortion for other reasons is contested.

Three passages from the Talmud—compiled in the sixth and seventh centuries—also figure prominently in later deliberation. One (from the tractate *Sanhedrin*) presents the opinion of Rav Huna that a minor may be considered a pursuer, or material aggressor, whose life may be taken in self-defense. Rav Ḥisda posed a question on the basis of the Mishnah. "We learned, 'once his head has come forth, he may not be harmed, for one may not set aside one life to save another.' But why so; is he not a pursuer?" The response: "There it is different, for she is pursued by heaven." A second passage (from *Arakhin*) discusses a situation that strikes modern readers as bizarre and most likely was never followed in practice. Although Talmudic authorities accepted capital punishment in principle, they believed that a delay between the imposition of a death sentence and the execution would represent cruel and unusual punishment for the guilty party. Accordingly, the Mishnah reports that if a pregnant woman is sentenced to death she is executed immediately. The Talmud reports the view of Samuel, as quoted by Rav Judah, that the fetus is killed before the execution "so that she will not be subject to disgrace (*nivul*)." Although this ruling has no direct practical application today, some authorities have cited this precedent to allow abortion to prevent anguish or shame. A third passage (again from *Sanhedrin*) presents the midrash (creative exegesis) of Rabbi Ishmael on Genesis 9:6. This passage generally is understood to mean, "Whoever sheds the blood of man, by man shall his blood be shed." The Hebrew also could be read, "Whoever sheds the blood of man in man, his blood shall be shed." The "man in man" is identified as the fetus in the mother's womb. Accordingly, at least generally and in principle, abortion would be a capital offense.[16]

Two passages from medieval authorities have been understood to pull in opposite directions in the abortion debate. The first is from the commentary of Rashi (eleventh century), explaining the rulings of the first Talmudic passage concerning innocent aggressors: "For as long as it has not come into the world it is not a living person (*nefesh*) and it is permissible to take its life in order to save its mother. Once the head has come forth one may not touch it to kill it, for then it is considered born, and one life may not be taken to save another." This passage would tend to support an understanding of a lesser status for the fetus. Another passage is found in the legal code of Moses Maimonides (twelfth century), the *Mishneh Torah*. "This is, moreover, a mitzvah (commandment), not to take pity on the life of a pursuer. Therefore, the sages have ruled that if a woman has difficulty giving birth, one dismembers the fetus within her womb, either by drugs or by surgery, because it is like a pursuer seeking to kill her. Once its head has emerged, it may not be touched, for we do not set aside one life for another; this is the natural course of the world." Many later thinkers have understood this passage to reflect a status for the fetus at least virtually equivalent to that of the mother—with relatively restrictive implications for abortion.[17]

As summarized by David Feldman, later authorities generally may be categorized into two groups, both agreeing that although abortion generally is prohibited it does not constitute homicide and that it is permitted to save the woman's life. One group follows Maimonides, regarding the fetus as having almost the full status of a human person and abortion as akin to homicide. These authorities may "build down" from this position, ruling leniently by construing threats to the woman's life broadly. The other group follows Rashi, emphasizing the subordinate status of the fetus, but then "builds up" to avoid indiscriminate abortion.[18] Rabbi Joseph Trani (Maharit, seventeenth century) was responsible for perhaps the first responsum dealing with elective abortion. He held that the fetus is not a *nefesh*, so abortion does not constitute homicide, but that abortion represents a generally impermissible wounding of the woman. Abortion is permitted "for need" or for the mother's healing. Rabbi Yair Bachrach (seventeenth century) understood abortion to violate a prohibition against contraception (or "wasting seed"). Although this position could allow room for exceptions for compelling reasons, Bachrach refused permission for a woman experiencing remorse after adultery, to avoid condoning and fostering immorality. Rabbi Jacob Emden (eighteenth century) understood abortion to violate a prohibition against contraception. He cautiously found room to permit abortion in a case of a woman who was pregnant from an adulterous relationship. "There is room for leniency for great need, as long as the birth process has not started, even if it is not to save the life of the mother, but to save her from the evil of great pain." For authorities such as Ezekiel Landau (eighteenth century) and Ḥayim Soloveitchik (nineteenth century), however, the status of the fetus is virtually equal to that of the mother. Abortion is permitted only to save her life, justified only by the pursuer argument in conjunction with the slightly lesser status of the fetus. Abortion in other cases would violate the prohibition against homicide.[19]

Status of the Fetus or Unborn Child

Personhood

For most Catholic writers the fetus should be considered an unborn child, to be respected as a human person, with the same right to life as all other human persons. The overwhelming majority of Catholic thinkers endorse this status for a fetus beyond the first two weeks of development. This position has been powerfully affirmed by the magisterium. In a 1951 allocution Pope Pius XII proclaimed, "The baby in the maternal breast has the right to life immediately from God. . . . The baby, still not born, is a man in the same degree and for the same reason as the mother." Likewise, Ashley and O'Rourke write that the unborn child "is a human person endowed with a spiritual soul and therefore endowed with the same human rights as any adult person. Its rights cannot be placed in competition with those of the mother, because both have the same basis and are equally to be respected."[20]

Even some thinkers who advocate a somewhat more liberal stance toward abortion than does the magisterium would agree that the unborn child (at least through most of pregnancy) has the same status as other human persons. Richard McCormick includes as "human life" "human life from fertilization or at least from the time" of individuation—about two weeks after conception. Although human life—whether that of an adult or that of an unborn child—may be taken in some cases of conflict, such compromises of the right to life are equally difficult to justify for the unborn child as for an adult or born child. "The best way to state why I share the traditional evaluation," McCormick writes, "is that I can think of no persuasive arguments that limit the sanctity of human life to extrauterine life. In other words, arguments that justify abortion seem to me equally to justify infanticide—and more."[21] Similarly Charles Curran writes, "On the question of the beginning of human life I see great wisdom in the teaching of the hierarchical magisterium of the Catholic Church and modify it only to the extent of placing the beginning of truly individual human life at two or three weeks after conception." Curran argues for the acceptance of some abortion not by claiming that the status of uterine life is lower than that of extrauterine but by arguing on the basis of both tradition and reason for greater flexibility in conflict situations.[22]

No Jewish authority considers the status of the fetus to be fully equal to that of the mother, even at the end of gestation. This position appears to be motivated in part by the traditional authority of the Mishnah text and in part by the dominant value of saving life (the woman's) reflected in that text. Some Jewish thinkers do accord the fetus the value of a person, virtually equivalent (though not quite fully equivalent) to that of the mother. Rabbis Ḥayim Soloveitchik and Mosheh Feinstein rule that the fetus is a person (*nefesh*), though not yet fully so (*nefesh gamur*). Because of this status, and because the fetus's future viability is less certain than that of the mother, abortion would be permitted when that is the only way to save the mother's life. Otherwise, however, abortion would represent the killing of a person and hence would be prohibited as homicide.[23]

Some Catholic writers, along with most Jewish writers, argue that the fetus (at least in early stages) does not have the status of a person. Nonetheless, it represents human life that has the potential to become a person. As such, it should be accorded significant value, and ending its life would be wrong *prima facie* (that is, unless required by a competing and compelling moral responsibility). Catholic thinkers who attribute personhood to the fetus only after a certain stage of development still accord significant status, short of personhood, to the earlier fetus. Catholic thinker Lisa Sowle Cahill writes:

> I am convinced that the fetus is from conception a member of the human species (having an identifiably human genotype, and being of human parentage), and, as such, is an entity to which at least some protection is due, even though its status may not at every phase be equivalent to that of postnatal life. . . . I see the fetus as having a value at conception that is quite significant and that quickly increases; but it never overrides the right of the mother to preserve her own life.[24]

Likewise Conservative rabbis Ben Zion Bokser and Kassel Abelson write, "The fetus is a life in the process of development, and the decision to abort it should never be taken lightly."[25] Some Jewish writers argue that current scientific understanding supports a higher status for the fetus than that found in some traditional sources—close to if not quite equal to personhood.[26] Others emphasize that abortion destroys "potential life," prevents the development of a personal life of observing *mitzvot* (commandments), and contradicts the creative work of God.[27]

Stages of Development

According to the magisterium and many Catholic theologians, the fetus must be respected as having the full status of personhood from the time of conception. As expressed in the "Declaration on Procured Abortion":

> Respect for human life is called for from the time that the process of generation begins. From the time that the ovum is fertilized, a life is begun which is neither that of the father nor of the mother; it is rather the life of a new human being with his own growth. It would never be made human if it were not already.[28]

This document and others argue that contemporary science has corroborated the status of full personal life for even the earliest "fruit of human generation," from the time of conception.[29] Ashley and O'Rourke emphasize the continuity of the individual, from syngamy (the formation of a single nucleus in the zygote) through birth and beyond. From the very beginning the zygote has not only a unique genome but "an active potentiality for self-development."[30]

Several Catholic thinkers have raised questions regarding the status of the zygote and embryo during the first two weeks of development. For much of this time the embryo can divide into twins because individual cells are totipotent—capable of becoming varied sorts of tissues and even an independent embryo. It also is possible for two embryos to combine to form into one. Moreover, the earliest embryo does not yet have any specialization of cells or internal structure. For John Mahoney, these considerations "indicate that, rather than ensoulment occurring at the stage of conception, it can take place only when there is an unambiguously individual subject capable of receiving the soul by virtue of the fact that it is passing beyond the stage of simple reduplication and is beginning to ramify and diversify through the development of its bodily organs."[31]

Other thinkers, such as Ashley and O'Rourke, respond that the strongest evidence supports personhood from the time of conception. The phenomenon of twinning is not decisive; when twinning occurs, one of the twins represents the continuation of the original individual and the other a new individual who comes into existence at the time of separation. Even the earliest embryo has significant internal organization. Ashley and O'Rourke state that "it is at the least highly probable" that this status of full and equal personhood applies from the time of conception.[32]

Ashley and O'Rourke do acknowledge that some considerations support the view that the earliest embryo may not yet be a person (even if the preponderance of the evidence supports personhood). The magisterium traditionally has been reluctant to claim absolute certainty regarding the moment of ensoulment. Although the "Declaration on Procured Abortion" asserts that human life begins at conception and must be fully respected, it does not claim to resolve "the question of the moment when the spiritual soul is infused. There is not a unanimous tradition on this point and authors are as yet in disagreement." Such theoretical discussions "have no bearing" on the practical duty to safeguard the life of the developing entity from the moment of conception. First, even before ensoulment, there would be "nothing less than a human life, preparing for and calling for a soul." Second, even if the status of the earliest embryo were uncertain, this uncertainty would require absolute protection of its life. "From a moral point of view this is certain: even if a doubt existed concerning whether the fruit of conception is already a human person, it is objectively a grave sin to dare to risk murder."[33]

Thinkers such as Mahoney respond that although the possibility of personhood must be taken seriously, it is not necessarily decisive. One must consider how likely it is that the early embryo is a person and the strength of considerations that argue for the ending of its life. Because it is unlikely that the earliest embryo is a person, its death could be justified by compelling reasons. Nevertheless, its status, though not that of a person, remains significant. "The unensouled fetus has promise. . . . What is in preparation is the body as temple of the Holy Spirit and the human person imaged after God and befriended by his all-encompassing love," Mahoney writes. Although destruction of the fetus may not be homicide, "even in the very earliest days . . . such an action could not responsibly be undertaken for any but most the serious reasons." Similarly, McCormick writes that although the preembryo is not a person, it has the intrinsic potential to become one. "I would argue that the preembryo should be treated as a person but that this is a *prima facie* obligation only."[34]

A few Catholic thinkers have suggested that personhood may not begin until a later stage of development. Some note that a human person is a rational entity. Such an entity could not exist without a minimal physical structure that could support rationality. Thinkers suggest as key points of development the beginnings of the cerebral cortex structure by about forty days, the development of major systems and initial neural activity by about eight weeks, and the integration of the nervous system about the twentieth week.[35] Most Catholic writers, however, argue that such milestones represent quantitative rather than qualitative changes that do not alter the status of the fetus. Few Catholic theologians have advocated relational criteria for personhood, arguing that the fetus should not be considered a person until it is accepted as such by parents or society, which may not occur until late in pregnancy; this view is overwhelmingly rejected by a wide range of thinkers.[36] Although a few thinkers have held that the fetus does not become a person until birth, no major theologian currently advocates this view.[37]

In contrast, all Jewish writers agree that the fetus does not fully acquire the status of personhood until birth.[38] Nevertheless, most hold that the fetus does have a significant status that generally would prohibit abortion, albeit with exceptions in appropriate cases. Some Jewish writers have suggested various stages as representing changes in the fetus's status, rendering abortion somewhat easier to justify early in gestation and more difficult to justify in later stages. The Talmud refers to the embryo before forty days of development as "mere fluid" (corresponding roughly with much Catholic ancient and medieval thought). For some authorities, this status suggests greater leeway for abortion in the earliest stages. Perceptible fetal movement is understood to occur after about three months of gestation. One contemporary authority refers to viability, at about six months, as a significant marker. Generally, however, these stages are understood to represent quantitative change—somewhat altering the strength of reasons needed to justify abortion but not decisively altering fetal status. Even at the earliest stages, fetal status is significant, requiring compelling reasons to justify abortion; even at the last stages before birth, the fetus does not have an equal status to the mother.[39]

Prohibition of Abortion and Possible Exceptions

Absolute Prohibition

For the Catholic magisterium, the prohibition against abortion is absolute. As expressed in the U.S. bishops' "Ethical and Religious Directives": "Abortion, that is, the directly intended termination of pregnancy before viability or the directly intended destruction of a viable fetus, is never permitted." As I have noted, Pope Pius XI asserts that although one has sympathy for a woman whose health and even life are threatened by a continuation of the pregnancy, this sympathy would not justify murder—which is what abortion would represent. Indeed, in the late nineteenth century the Holy Office explicitly condemned views allowing abortion when the alternative was the death of both mother and child.[40] More recently, the "Declaration on Procured Abortion" proclaims:

> The gravity of the problem comes from the fact that in certain cases, perhaps in quite a considerable number of cases, by denying abortion one endangers important values which men normally hold in great esteem and which may sometimes even seem to have priority. We do not deny these very great difficulties. It may be a serious question of health, sometimes of life or death, for the mother. . . . We proclaim only that none of these reasons can ever objectively confer the right to dispose of another's life, even when that life is only beginning.[41]

Ashley and O'Rourke endorse the absolute prohibition of abortion: "The direct killing of innocent human beings can never be justifiable." They argue that this commitment does not entail simple acceptance of the mother's death. With contemporary medical developments, the physician is able to seek to save both mother and child or at least attempt to save the mother without directly choosing to end the life of the child. They also note the magisterial acceptance of some "indirect" abortions, justified by the principle of double effect. "An indirect abortion is one in which the direct, immediate purpose of the procedure is to treat the mother for some threatening pathology, but in which the death of the fetus is an inevitable result that would have been avoided had it been possible." A classic example is the removal of a cancerous uterus from a pregnant woman. This action is justified in part because the removal of the uterus directly helps her, and the death of the fetus is an unintended side effect.[42] The removal of a fallopian tube from a woman with an ectopic pregnancy has long been accepted on similar grounds. As classically argued by T. Lincoln Bouscaren, in such a case the tube could be considered pathological and removed on that basis, with the death of the embryo an unintended side effect. More recently, John F. Tuohey has argued for the acceptability of an operation to remove a trophoblast containing an embryo from a fallopian tube. Ashley and O'Rourke have argued more generally for the acceptability of removing an embryo from a fallopian tube, considering this position to be consistent with the U.S. bishops' general guidance: "In case of extrauterine pregnancy, no intervention is morally licit which constitutes a direct abortion."[43]

Abortion to Save the Mother's Life

Germain Grisez has advocated a further expansion of procedures that may be considered indirect. He suggests a revised understanding of the principle of double effect, in which different effects of an action may be considered to be equally immediate. In cases in which abortion is required to save the mother's life, the death of the child is not intended; the removal of the child from the mother is sought, with the inevitable consequence (given current medical technology) that the child will die. This death could be regarded as an unintended side effect of the abortion, which could be justified to preserve the mother's life.

> This justification will also apply to abortions previously considered direct having strict medical indications such as those mentioned involving impaired heart and/or kidney function. The justification is simply that the very same act, indivisible as to its behavioral process, has both the good effect of protecting human life and the bad effect of destroying it. The fact that the good effect is subsequent in time and in physical process to the evil one is irrelevant, because the entire process is indivisible by human choice and hence all aspects of it are equally present to the agent at the moment he makes his choice.[44]

All Jewish thinkers would accept abortion if required to save the mother's life. This permission partly reflects Jewish understandings regarding the status of the fetus, allowing for greater leniency with regard to ending the life of the fetus. It also reflects the power of the imperative to preserve life (see in chapters 2 and 4), entailing stringency in this regard. For example, Orthodox rabbi Immanuel Jakobovits condemns abortion as "an appurtenance of murder" and argues against abortion in cases involving rape or likely birth defects. He advocates national laws restricting abortion, even if these restrictions impose suffering in some cases. Nevertheless, abortion to prevent a threat to the mother's life is mandated. Indeed, "such a threat to the mother need not be either immediate or absolutely certain. Even a remote risk of life invokes all the life-saving concessions of Jewish law, provided the fear of such a risk is genuine and confirmed by the most competent medical opinions. Hence, Jewish law would regard it as an indefensible desecration of human life to allow a mother to perish in order to save her unborn child."[45] Some other Jewish thinkers would agree that abortion is permitted only to save the mother's life. Abortion for any other reason would be condemned as unjustifiable homicide.[46]

Abortion to Avoid Serious Threats to Health

Some Catholic thinkers would cautiously expand the range of legitimate abortion to include not only threats to the mother's life but also some other serious threats to the health and well-being of the mother or others. Bernard Häring suggests room for expansion of the scope of indirect abortion: "Many moralists of past centuries spoke on indirect abortion in a very broad sense. Their teaching was applied in one way or another to almost all cases where the chief and decisive intention was directed toward another good—the health and life of the mother." Interventions that end the life of the fetus in such cases avoid the characteristic "malice of abortion" and therefore need not be severely condemned.[47]

Other Catholic writers, instead of broadening the category of indirect abortions, challenge the significance accorded to the distinction between direct and indirect. Richard McCormick argues that fetal life may be ended only for reasons that would justify ending the life of born persons. Such an action "may be taken only when doing so is the only life-saving and life-serving alternative, or when doing so is, all things considered (not just the numbers) the lesser evil. . . . For an act to be life-saving and life-serving, to be the lesser evil (all things considered), there must be at stake human life or its moral equivalent, a good or a value comparable to life itself." Because humans go to war to preserve freedom (and are permitted by the tradition to do so), freedom is one such value comparable to life. Accordingly, abortion could be allowed when it is necessary to avoid insanity for the mother when that condition would entail "complete and permanent loss of freedom."[48] Similarly, Charles Curran argues that the values at stake, rather than an act's physical structure of causality, must be decisive in formulating a moral evaluation. "Abortion can be justified for preserving the life of the mother and for other important values commensurate with life even though the action aims at abortion as a means to an end." Such reasons could include preventing "very grave psychological or physical harm to the mother with the realization that this must truly be grave harm that will perdure over some time and not just a temporary depression."[49] Although Lisa Sowle Cahill does not equate the life of a fetus with that of born persons, she agrees that only the most compelling reasons could justify abortion: "Threat to life is the classic case," she writes, "although I would not exclude the possibility that other threats might justify abortion, particularly when the interest that the mother has at stake is equal to or greater than her interest in her life."[50]

Most Jewish writers would agree with these Catholic thinkers in accepting abortion in some cases that do not involve immediate threat to the woman's life. Reflecting the values and precedents of the tradition, they tend to do so by expansively construing the mandate to prevent threats to life. Most authorities consider severe psychiatric illness as potentially representing a danger to life, so even some authorities who generally oppose abortion would authorize it in some cases to avoid such dangers.[51] Many would allow abortion to avoid a severe threat to the woman's health, even when her life is not endangered; they argue that abortion does not represent homicide, nor is it biblically forbidden—so the prohibition of abortion may be superseded by the imperative of healing.[52] A consensus statement of the Conservative movement's Committee on Jewish Law and Standards holds that "abortion is justifiable if a continuation of the pregnancy might cause the mother severe physical or psychological harm."[53]

Orthodox rabbi Ben Zion Uziel allowed abortion in a case in which the woman was threatened by deafness from a continuation of the pregnancy. Although this case involved medical risk, Uziel offers a more general rationale for permissible abortion. He cites the Talmud's authorization of fetal death to save a woman from emotional anguish (in connection with capital punishment), as well as Emden's acceptance of abortion following adultery for "great need" and to save the woman from "great pain." Uziel continues, "It is clear that abortion is not permitted unless there is a need, even a slim need (*tzorekh kalush*) such as avoiding dishonor for the mother, but it is certain that if there is no need it is forbidden, because of destruction and the prevention of the possibility of life."[54] Writing about this opinion, Feldman uses language very similar to that in Catholic thinkers such as McCormick: "The law of Israel, just as it requires that the foetus be sacrificed to save the mother's physical life, likewise requires that it be sacrificed to save her spirit from torture and suffering."[55]

Abortion for Other Reasons

Uziel's argument for abortion to avoid maternal deafness suggests a broader range of reasons that might be invoked to justify abortion. Abortion could be justified for great need or to avoid suffering and shame, even without invoking medical threat. Relatively few Catholic thinkers advocate expansion of justifications for abortion beyond avoidance of direct threats to the mother's health. Daniel Maguire argues that Christian prolife commitments, properly understood, support abortion in appropriate circumstances. "Abortion is justified only when it promotes life in its complex reality and balance. In an example that should be obvious, the poor woman who chooses abortion because she cannot feed adequately the children she already has is making a pro-life decision."[56] A group of theologians led by Bruno Ribes accepts abortion in extreme cases, not limited to medical threat. "No abortion situation is 'socially justifiable' unless accompanied by an attestation of the impossibility for the parents to give birth without creating an inhuman situation."[57] Christine Gudorf argues that although people are called to undergo some degree of sacrifice to help others, there are limits to moral obligation. "No one should ever sacrifice her essential self—which is not reducible to physical life—in the interest of the fetus or any other life." Abortion would be justified if threats to the woman's health or "serious defect in the fetus" would otherwise make her life "insupportable." For some women and in some cases, threats to the woman's chosen career or to her personal relationships could suffice to justify abortion, to preserve her essential self. In addition, Gudorf raises the possibility that "population pressure" might justify abortion in some circumstances.[58]

Many Jewish authorities accept abortion in some circumstances to avoid suffering by the woman, even when her health is not directly threatened. Abortion of a fetus with a serious genetic disease, such as Tay-Sachs disease, often is approached in these terms. Jewish writers typically do not claim that the future suffering of the child after birth would make his or her life not worth living; instead, they justify such abortion when it would save the woman from anguish that she would find unbearable. Orthodox rabbi Eliezer Yehudah Waldenberg, for example, appeals to Emden's acceptance of abortion for great need and to avoid great pain. "If so, ask yourself if there is need, suffering, and pain greater than that of our case" involving prenatal diagnosis of Tay-Sachs; as the child suffered on the way to certain death within a number of years, the parents would suffer the anguish of observing without being able to help. This scenario would represent a clear case of allowing abortion for great need and to avoid suffering. Waldenberg expresses greater hesitancy about aborting a fetus with less severe problems. Generally, a fetus with Down syndrome should not be aborted. Indeed, Waldenberg urges a questioner to avoid amniocentesis to test for this condition because that procedure would entail unnecessary wounding to the woman and risk fetal death. Amniocentesis would be appropriate only when the husband or wife is consumed with worry, unable to sleep day or night. Similarly, aborting a fetus with Down syndrome could be acceptable only in exceptional circumstances—when there is great need because giving birth to a child with this condition would lead to anguish, illness, and harm to the marriage. Such permission could be given cautiously and on a case-by-case basis only, with the authorization of a rabbi who is familiar with the specific circumstances involved.[59]

Other rabbis, arguing along similar lines, are somewhat more willing to accept abortion in cases of fetal deformity. Conservative rabbi Kassel Abelson writes, "If the tests indicate that the child will be born with major defects that would preclude a normal life and that make the mother and the family anxious about the future, it is permitted to abort the fetus."[60] Similarly, Reform rabbi Solomon Freehof asserts that in a case in which a pregnant woman had been exposed to rubella—entailing a likelihood of physical and mental deformity in the fetus—"then for the mother's sake (i.e., her mental anguish now and in the future)" abortion may be performed.[61]

Blu Greenberg is willing to stretch the rubric of therapeutic abortion even further; although she is an Orthodox layperson, her views differ markedly from those of Orthodox rabbinic authorities. Greenberg acknowledges halakhic precedent restricting abortion, as well as dangers of abuse and the devaluation of life, but also notes competing values. "Unless one is physically and emotionally unable to cope, not yet settled in marriage, etc., abortion should be avoided." Precedents allowing abortion to guard the woman's psychological health could be expanded to "encompass such variables as physical strength, stress, even delay in child-raising for purposes of family planning or a career." Like Gudorf, Greenberg understands herself as a feminist who is part of a religious community and informed by traditional values; also like Gudorf, Greenberg advocates allowing women to choose abortion when compelled by personal needs and concern for family relationships.[62]

Reform rabbi Balfour Brickner advocates a broad scope for a woman's right to choose abortion, expressing less hesitancy and ambivalence than does Greenberg. He emphasizes that the tradition does not consider the fetus a person, so the value of the woman's autonomy is decisive. Brickner understands this stance to support women's right to choose abortion without restrictions as a matter of U.S. law and deference to individual conscience and women's choices as a matter of morality. He expresses views similar to those of Maguire, although in more extreme form.

> It is precisely because of this regard for that sanctity [of human life] that we see as most desirable the right of any couple to be free to produce only that number of children whom they feel they could feed and clothe and educate properly: only that number to whom they could devote themselves as real parents, as creative partners with God. It is precisely this traditional Jewish respect for the sanctity of human life that moves us now to support that legislation which would help all women to be free to choose when and under what circumstances they would choose to bring life into the world.[63]

Even Brickner, at the prochoice extreme on the spectrum of Jewish writers, acknowledges a need for thoughtfulness in making moral decisions about abortion. "Jewish law teaches a reverent and responsible attitude to the question of abortion," he writes. "Judaism looks on abortion with distaste, discourages and tries to restrict it, but it clearly permits it."[64] Other Jewish writers—Reform and Conservative as well as Orthodox—give greater emphasis to moral concerns weighing against abortion. Many take care to distinguish their liberal stance from simple abortion on demand. As one Reform responsum concludes, "We do not encourage abortion, nor favor it for trivial reasons, or sanction it 'on demand.'" Likewise, a consensus statement from the Conservative Rabbinical Assembly proclaims, "Jewish tradition is sensitive to the sanctity of life and does not permit abortion on demand."[65]

Pastoral Sensitivity and Societal Concerns

Many of the Catholic writers who adamantly proclaim that abortion is morally wrong in all instances note the possibility of more flexible judgments regarding individual guilt in particular cases. Even Pope John Paul II's *Gospel of Life*, a forceful and absolute condemnation of abortion and other sins against life, offers such possibilities. A woman might choose abortion "out of a desire to protect certain important values such as her own health or a decent standard of living for the other members of the family." "Decisions that go against life sometimes arise from difficult or even tragic situations. . . . Such circumstances can mitigate even to a notable degree subjective responsibility and the consequent culpability of those who make these choices which in themselves are evil."[66] Ashley and O'Rourke insist that their concern is focused on the objective wrongness of abortion, not the subjective culpability of individuals who choose abortion in admittedly difficult circumstances. "It may seem contrary to the command of Jesus, 'Do not judge, and you will not be judged,' for Christians to condemn as murderers such women and the compassionate physicians who assist them. Yes, instead of judgment, Christians must seek ways to assist women to escape such anguishing dilemmas."[67]

McCormick reports a similar stance in his review of statements from European bishops. "While urging the teaching [against abortion] clearly and unflinchingly, the bishops manifest a great compassion for individuals in tragic circumstances and a refusal to judge these individuals." McCormick argues for the importance of combining a stringent and prophetic declaration of general moral norms with compassionate consideration of particular cases.[68] Bernard Häring emphasizes the greater flexibility appropriate to pastoral counseling in particular circumstances. He considers a case of pregnancy following rape. Abortion would not be morally acceptable. "Nevertheless, we must recognize that although the fetus is innocent, the girl is likewise innocent. We can therefore understand her revulsive feeling that this is not 'her' child, not a child that she is in justice required to bear. We must, however, try to motivate her to consider the child with love. . . . If, owing to the psychological effects of her traumatic experience, she is utterly unable to accept this counsel, it is possible that we may have to leave her in 'invincible ignorance.'" Häring would not positively recommend abortion. "But during the pastoral counselling I would refrain from all rigid judgment once I could see that the person cannot bear the burden of a clear appeal not to abort."[69] Although Häring is careful to distinguish between moral and pastoral analysis, he also suggests that, at least for practical purposes, his nuanced position differs little from a simple moral acceptance of abortion in appropriate cases.[70]

McCormick reports that accompanying European bishops' compassion for individual women "there is a rather persistent severity with society in general, whose conditions so often render new births difficult or psychologically insupportable." He notes a "unanimous and strongly stated conviction of the episcopates that we must do much more, personally and societally, to get at the causes of abortion."[71] Pope John Paul II casts the net of blame for abortion widely, including the unborn child's father, friends and family of the woman, and health care professionals who perform abortions. Also at fault are "those who have encouraged the spread of an attitude of sexual permissiveness and a lack of esteem for motherhood, and . . . those who should have ensured— but did not—effective family and social policies in support of families."[72] The "Declaration on Procured Abortion" states:

> It is the task of law to pursue a reform of society and of conditions
> of life in all milieux, starting with the most deprived, so that always
> and everywhere it may be possible to give every child coming into

this world a welcome worthy of a person. Help for families and for unmarried mothers, assured grants for children, legislation for illegitimate children and reasonable arrangements for adoption—a whole positive policy must be put into force so that there will always be a concrete honourable and possible alternative to abortion. . . . One can never approve of abortion; but it is above all necessary to combat its causes.[73]

Writers across the spectrum of Catholic thought agree on the need to address causes of abortion, as well as the importance of material and social support for families and expectant mothers. Häring recommends that "there should be more intelligent efforts to remove the chief causes of abortion and to enlighten public opinion about the whole problem."[74] Lisa Sowle Cahill concurs with the importance of education and support. "Needed to end abortion are deep changes in women's self-image and opportunities. . . . Young women need a sense of self-respect and adequate control over their own circumstances." Like the magisterium, Cahill challenges societal attitudes of individualism and sexual irresponsibility. "My practical approach to abortion is to counter 'abortion on demand' with better educational and social efforts to avoid unwanted pregnancy and to make the choice to give birth realistically available when unplanned pregnancy does occur."[75] Daniel Maguire argues that "the most intelligent way to be anti-abortion is to look to the causes of unwanted pregnancies." His list of causes to be combated resembles those identified by thinkers who are more absolute in their opposition to abortion. These causes include sexism, poverty, and the prevalence of a superficial "cult of romantic love." "The Judeo-Christian treasure houses a notion of love that could lead to more respectful relationships and more reverent sexual mores and fewer and fewer women at the clinic door."[76]

Although Jewish writers tend to devote less extensive discussion to factors that lead to abortion, some express concerns similar to those of their Catholic counterparts. For example, Immanuel Jakobovits criticizes sexual irresponsibility. He also insists that society do more "to assume the burdens which the individual family can no longer bear."[77] Blu Greenberg shares many views with Catholic writers who are much more restrictive regarding the morality of abortion. She advocates greater sexual responsibility and worries about "the devaluation of human life." "Abortion is really a symptom of a larger problem. Ours is a society which establishes the value of goods over relationships, or possessions over people, or ease and comfort over labor and a life of giving. . . . As a result, contemporary society borders on the selfish."[78]

Conclusion

At the level of abstract principle, Jewish and Roman Catholic writers disagree dramatically about the status of the fetus or unborn child. For most Catholics, the unborn child must be respected as a person, starting at a point no later than a few weeks after conception. For Jews, the fetus must be respected as potential personal life but does not have the full status of a person even in the last weeks of gestation. At the level of practical norms and moral decision making, however, the difference is far less sharp. As with life-sustaining treatment (see chapter 4), Jewish and Catholic positions on abortion represent overlapping spectra, though with the Catholic spectrum now extending to the right. According to the magisterium and many individual Catholic theologians, direct abortion is never licit, even to save the mother's life. Many Catholic writers and all Jewish writers would permit abortion when necessary to save the mother's life. Most Jewish authorities and some of their Catholic counterparts would permit abortion to avoid a serious threat to the mother's health, and many Jewish thinkers would accept abortion in some other circumstances to avoid significant personal suffering for the mother. Some Catholic writers would accept abortion in some such cases; a larger number would express some acceptance of decisions for abortion at the pastoral level—understanding a woman who chooses abortion following the trauma of rape, for example, not to be culpable.

Lisa Sowle Cahill articulates the common ground among diverse Catholic thinkers: "To use the labels of convenience, both liberal/progressive and conservative/traditionalist Catholics tend generally to see life at all stages as having significant value, to see abortion on demand as a bad thing, to see other alternatives as far preferable and to think that these views are philosophically and humanistically defensible."[79] Jewish thinkers overwhelmingly would share these points of consensus. Similarly, Bernard Häring emphasizes areas of agreement between

Catholic and Protestant thinkers: "To my knowledge, Protestant writers affirm unambiguously the same basic moral values as those on which we ground our own argumentation; there is therefore a broad agreement about the immorality of abortion in general. Disagreement arises chiefly about hard cases where Protestants hold that, because of special circumstances, other moral values dominate in such a way that what is still called abortion does not show the specific malice of abortion."[80] The same appraisal would hold in comparing Catholic and Jewish writers.[81]

Jewish writers tend to agree with Catholics on the importance of addressing factors that are among the causes of abortion. Poverty and sexism should be fought. Greater support should be provided to women, children, and families. Attitudes and practices reflecting respect for human life and sexual responsibility should be fostered. A joint statement of Jews and Catholics from Los Angeles provides one example of shared goals. These goals include

> advocacy of positive alternatives to abortion and promotion of social situations which will encourage the responsible bearing and rearing of children:
> a. Strengthening of families. . . .
> b. Healing for broken families and assistance to parents who are raising their children alone.
> c. Counseling and assistance during pregnancy especially for the unmarried.
> d. Guidance toward adoption services for mothers unable to care for children.
> e. Instruction in parenting and child-raising.
> f. Nurture of stable and caring families.

The statement concludes, "While Roman Catholics and Jews may not agree to make the prohibition of all abortions American law, nonetheless we should work together to make respect for life, and particularly the joyful celebration of new life, an American ideal."[82]

Although one must acknowledge similarities of Jewish and Roman Catholic approaches to abortion, the differences between the traditions remain noteworthy. The roots of this divergence reach back to the Bible. For traditional Judaism, the Torah represents the paradigmatic revelation of God's will and serves as the foundational text for ascertaining concrete moral responsibilities. The clear distinction between the status of woman and fetus in Exodus 21 provides a touchstone for the subsequent development of Jewish law and ethics; this distinction is reaffirmed in the Mishnah and subsequent sources. Early Christianity was more strongly influenced by the Septuagint; the rendering of this passage there supports the equal status of the unborn child after formation with the woman. In addition, Christianity has accorded special esteem to the prophetic books within the Hebrew Bible. Passages such as that reflecting God's relationship with Jeremiah in the womb could exert greater influence than Toraitic law. For Judaism, prophetic books have hortatory and inspirational value but less readily provide the grounding for specific obligations. Most dramatically distinguishing biblical influences on Christianity and Judaism are the infancy narratives of the New Testament, with John the Baptist joyfully responding to Jesus while both were in utero.[83]

Another historical divergence between the two traditions concerns contraception. For many thinkers in each tradition, the prohibition against abortion has been strongly linked to that against contraception. This link was clear in ancient sources and has continued for some thinkers at least into the twentieth century. Historically, for some thinkers the prohibition of abortion (at least early in gestation) derives simply from that against contraception, and the prohibition of contraception is at least as stringent as that regarding abortion.[84] The dominant position in Catholic thought has been an absolute prohibition of contraception. The dominant Jewish position has been that contraception generally is prohibited but is mandated when needed to protect the life or health of a woman.[85] The paradigm of contraception would provide support for an absolute prohibition of abortion in Catholicism and a general prohibition of abortion that allows exceptions in Judaism. Although contraception is no longer central to arguments about abortion, it seems likely that this topic has had and continues to exert some influence.

One may gain a perspective on abortion by framing the issue in terms of the intrinsic dignity and value of human life, sometimes expressed as the sanctity of life. Each tradition is committed to this principle but specifies and balances this principle and others differently. For each tradition, the life and welfare of the pregnant woman has great value. For the magisterium and many Catholic thinkers, the life of the unborn child has equal value and is equally deserving of respect, so direct abortion is never acceptable. For Jewish thinkers the life of the fetus or unborn child has value and deserves respect, but somewhat less so than the woman. According to some authorities, the status of the fetus is virtually equal to that of the mother; commitment to the sanctity of life demands abortion to save the woman's life but condemns abortion in any other circumstance. For other Jewish thinkers, the imperative to preserve the life of the woman is construed more broadly, entailing a commitment to preserve the woman's health.[86] This approach reflects leniency with regard to fetal life but also the stringency to preserve life and health I discuss in chapter 4 and throughout this book. Yet other Jewish writers, along with some of their Catholic colleagues, emphasize that the sanctity of life and respect for human dignity involve more than safeguarding biological existence. There are limits to the sacrifice and suffering a pregnant woman is obligated to undergo, even to preserve the life of the fetus.

Adherents of both traditions agree on the important value of reverence for human life. One clear implication of this shared value is that, as a moral matter, abortion is at least *prima facie* wrong; that is, the moral prohibition against abortion is binding unless it is outweighed by competing ethical considerations. At the same time, reverence for human life supports attention to problems of poverty and attitudes of selfishness, which contribute to the prevalence of abortion and harm human well-being in many other ways.

Notes

1. Translations from the Hebrew Bible generally follow New Jewish Publication Society, *Tanakh* (Philadelphia: Jewish Publication Society, 1999) (NJPS). Translations from the New Testament follow *The New American Bible* with Revised New Testament (Washington, D.C.: Confraternity of Christian Doctrine, 1986) (NAB).

2. In John Connery, *Abortion: The Development of the Roman Catholic Perspective* (Chicago: Loyola University Press, 1977), 17; see also David M. Feldman, *Birth Control in Jewish Law*, rev. ed. (Northvale, N.J.: Jason Aronson, 1998), 257–58.

3. John T. Noonan suggests that condemnations of magical medicine (*pharmakeia*) may have been meant to include abortifacients, although John

Connery expresses doubt that abortion was the central concern in these passages. See Galatians 5:20, Revelation 9:21; John T. Noonan, "An Almost Absolute Value in History," in *The Morality of Abortion: Legal and Historical Perspectives*, ed. John T. Noonan (Cambridge: Harvard University Press, 1970), 8–9; Connery, *Abortion*, 34–35.

4. *Didache* 2.2, in Noonan, "Almost Absolute Value," 9.

5. Noonan, "Almost Absolute Value," 14–18; Connery, *Abortion*, 39–64.

6. This position was reflected in canon law under Pope Innocent III, as well as by authorities such as Gratian, Peter Lombard, and Thomas Aquinas. The decretals of Pope Gregory IX deemed all abortion, as well as contraception, to constitute homicide (Noonan, "Almost Absolute Value," 20–26; Connery, *Abortion*, 88–112).

7. *Quodlibeta* of John of Naples, in Noonan, "Almost Absolute Value," 26; Connery, *Abortion*, 115–16.

8. Connery, *Abortion*, 124–67; Noonan, "Almost Absolute Value," 27–32. For Sanchez, abortion of the early fetus is linked to contraception; in fact, the prohibition of contraception is more severe, less readily admitting exceptions than the prohibition of abortion (Noonan, "Almost Absolute Value," 28).

9. Noonan, "Almost Absolute Value," 35; Connery, *Abortion*, 168–72.

10. Noonan, "Almost Absolute Value," 34; Connery, *Abortion*, 189.

11. Connery, *Abortion*, 241, 220–69; Noonan, "Almost Absolute Value," 46–47.

12. Noonan, "Almost Absolute Value," 39; Connery, *Abortion*, 212. In 1588 Pope Sixtus V had applied the penalty of excommunication to all abortion, as well as contraception, but in 1591 Pope Gregory XIV restricted this penalty to abortion of the ensouled or animated fetus (Connery, *Abortion*, 148, Noonan, "Almost Absolute Value," 33).

13. Pius XI, *Casti Connubii: On Christian Marriage [CC]* (New York: Barry Vail, 1931), n. 64, pp. 29–30.

14. *Gaudium et Spes: Pastoral Constitution on the Church in the Modern World*, in *Vatican Council II: The Conciliar and Post Conciliar Documents*, new revised ed., ed. Austin Flannery (Northport, N.Y.: Costello, 1996), n. 51, p. 955; Noonan, "Almost Absolute Value," 44–46. In case of ectopic pregnancy, removal of the fallopian tube, but not the embryo, became accepted as consistent with the absolute prohibition of abortion, based on the principle of double effect. Removal of a cancerous uterus from a pregnant woman was similarly accepted (Noonan, "Almost Absolute Value," 47–50, Connery, *Abortion*, 295–303). See discussion below of indirect abortion.

15. Mishnah *Oholot* 7:6.

16. Talmud *Sanhedrin* 72b, *Arakhin* 7a, *Sanhedrin* 57b.

17. Rashi, commentary to *Sanhedrin* 72b; Maimonides, *Mishneh Torah*, "Laws of Murder and the Preservation of Life," 1:9.

18. Feldman, *Birth Control in Jewish Law*, 284.

19. Joseph Trani, *Resp. Maharit*, n. 99; Yair Bachrach, *Resp. Havot Ya'ir*, n. 31; Jacob Emden, *Resp. Sh'elat Ya'avetz*, n. 43; Ezekiel Landau, *Resp. Noda Bi'Yehudah, Mahadura Tinyana, Hoshen Mishpat*, n. 59; Hayim Soloveitchik, *Hiddushei R. Hayim Halevi al HaRambam* (Israel: n.p., 1992), commentary to Maimonides, *Mishneh Torah*, "Laws of Murder and the Preservation of Life," 1·9, pp. 266–67 (all discussed in Feldman, *Birth Control in Jewish Law*, 256–89); J. David Bleich, "Abortion in Halakhic Literature," in *Contemporary Halakhic Problems*, vol. 1 (New York: Ktav and Yeshiva University Press, 1977), 327–65; and Basil F. Herring, *Jewish Ethics and Halakhah for Our Time* (New York: Ktav and Yeshiva University Press, 1984), 31–43.

20. Pius XII, "Address to the Italian Catholic Society of Midwives," in Noonan, "Almost Absolute Value," 45; Benedict M. Ashley and Kevin D. O'Rourke, *Health Care Ethics: A Theological Analysis*, 4th ed. (Washington, D.C.: Georgetown University Press, 1997), 252.

21. Richard A. McCormick, "Public Policy on Abortion," in *How Brave a New World?* (Washington, D.C.: Georgetown University Press, 1981), 194–96.

22. Charles E. Curran, "Abortion: Ethical Aspects," in *Transition and Tradition in Moral Theology* (Notre Dame, Ind.: University of Notre Dame Press, 1979), 227. Curran argues (222) that "the accepted Catholic teaching allows less conflict situations for the fetus in the womb than for human life outside the womb" and that he is merely seeking to make the taking of fetal life no more difficult to justify than the taking of life of born persons. See also "The Fifth Commandment: Thou Shalt not Kill," in *Ongoing Revision: Studies in Moral Theology* (Notre Dame, Ind.: Fides, 1975), 153–58.

23. Soloveitchik, *Hiddushei R. Hayim Halevi al HaRambam*; Mosheh Feinstein, *Iggerot Moshe*, vol. 7 (Bnei Berak, Israel: Ohel Yosef, 1985), *Hoshen Mishpat* 2, n. 69, p. 296; and sources cited in Avraham Steinberg, *Encyclopedia of Jewish Medical Ethics*, vol. 2 (Jerusalem: Schlesinger Institute, 1988), s.v. "Abortion," 78–80.

24. Lisa Sowle Cahill, "Abortion, Autonomy, and Community," in *Abortion and Catholicism: The American Debate*, ed. Patricia Beattie Jung and Thomas A. Shannon (New York: Crossroad, 1988), 86.

25. Ben Zion Bokser and Kassel Abelson, "A Statement on the Permissibility of Abortion," in *Life and Death Responsibilities in Jewish Biomedical Ethics*, ed. Aaron L. Mackler (New York: Jewish Theological Seminary of America, Finkelstein Institute, 2000), 195.

26. David Novak, *Law and Theology in Judaism* (New York: Ktav, 1974), 123; Richard Alan Block, "The Right to Do Wrong: Reform Judaism and Abortion," *Journal of Reform Judaism* 28, no. 2 (1981): 9–12.

27. Isaac Klein, "A Teshuvah on Abortion," in Mackler, *Life and Death Responsibilities in Jewish Biomedical Ethics*, 208; Steinberg, *Encyclopedia of Jewish Medical Ethics*, vol. 2, 76–78.

28. "Declaration on Procured Abortion," in *Vatican Council II: More Postconciliar Documents*, ed. Austin Flannery (Collegeville, Minn.: Liturgical Press, 1982), n. 12, p. 445.

29. "Declaration on Procured Abortion," n. 13, p. 445; Congregation for the Doctrine of the Faith, *Donum Vitae: Instruction on Respect for Human Life in its Origin and on the Dignity of Procreation: Replies to Certain Questions of the Day* (Washington, D.C.: United States Catholic Conference, 1987), 12–14; John Paul II, *Evangelium Vitae: The Gospel of Life [EV]* (Washington, D.C.: United States Catholic Conference, 1995), n. 60, p. 107.

30. Ashley and O'Rourke, *Health Care Ethics*, 230–32.

31. John Mahoney, *Bioethics and Belief* (London: Sheed and Ward, 1984), 67. See similarly Charles Curran, "Abortion: Its Legal and Moral Aspects in Catholic Theology," in *New Perspectives in Moral Theology* (Notre Dame, Ind.: University of Notre Dame Press, 1976), 188–89; Richard A. McCormick, "Who or What Is the Preembryo?" *Kennedy Institute of Ethics Journal* 1 (1991): 8–13; Thomas A. Shannon and Allan B. Wolter, "Reflections on the Moral Status of the Pre-embryo," *Theological Studies* 51 (1990): 610–14; Lisa Sowle Cahill, "The Embryo and the Fetus: New Moral Contexts," *Theological Studies* 54 (1993): 127–32; Bernard Häring, *Medical Ethics*, ed. Gabrielle L. Jean (Notre Dame, Ind.: Fides, 1973), 78–80, 101. Some authors also note that many early embryos naturally do not develop and that the process of development depends on information from the mother as well as from the fetus.

32. Ashley and O'Rourke, *Health Care Ethics*, 252, 227–40.

33. "Declaration on Procured Abortion," nn. 12–13, p. 446, and note 19, p. 452 (emphasis in original). Likewise Ashley and O'Rourke, *Health Care Ethics*, 252, assert, "It is at the least highly probable—and therefore in moral decisions practically certain—that from conception (syngamy) the human organism is a human person endowed with a spiritual soul and therefore endowed with the same human rights as any adult person."

34. Mahoney, *Bioethics and Belief*, 82–85; McCormick, "Who or What is the Preembryo?" 13. Shannon and Wolter articulate a similar view of early embryos in the first week or two of development, or "pre-embryos": "They possess ontic value and are in themselves valuable. . . . The pre-embryo at this state, we conclude, cannot claim absolute protection based on claims to per-

sonhood grounded in ontological individuality. Yet, since the pre-embryo is living and possesses genetic uniqueness, some claims to protection are possible. But these may not be absolute and, if not, could yield to other moral claims" ("Reflections on the Moral Status of the Pre-embryo," 624).

35. Shannon and Wolter, "Reflections on the Moral Status of the Pre-embryo," 622–24; Häring, *Medical Ethics*, 83–85.

36. See Curran, "Abortion: Ethical Aspects," 213–15; Richard McCormick, "Notes on Moral Theology: The Abortion Dossier," *Theological Studies* 35 (1974): 332–36.

37. See Connery's discussion of Baldus de Ubadis (*Abortion*, 102) and Ioannes Marcus (*Abortion*, 189).

38. Even an opponent of abortion such as Immanuel Jakobovits will acknowledge, "Jewish law assumes that the full title to life arises only at birth"; "Jewish Views on Abortion," in *Abortion and the Law*, ed. David T. Smith (Cleveland: Western Reserve University Press, 1967), 129.

39. See Feldman, *Birth Control in Jewish Law*, 265–67; Herring, *Jewish Ethics and Halakhah for Our Time*, 36–38; Eliezer Yehudah Waldenberg, *Tzitz Eliezer* (Jerusalem: n.p., 1985), v. 9, n. 51, section 3 (p. 239); v. 14, n. 100 (p. 186).

40. See National Conference of Catholic Bishops (NCCB), "Ethical and Religious Directives for Catholic Health Care Services," *Origins* 24 (1994), n. 45, p. 457; Pius XI, *CC*, 29–30; Noonan, "Almost Absolute Value," 41–43; and discussion above. Germain G. Grisez notes additional papal statements explicitly rejecting abortion, even to save the mother's life; see *Abortion: The Myths, the Realities, and the Arguments* (New York: Corpus, 1970), 181–82.

41. "Declaration on Procured Abortion," n. 14, p. 446. Pope John Paul II acknowledges that women sometimes choose abortion "out of a desire to protect certain important values such as her own health. . . . Nevertheless, these reasons and others like them, however serious and tragic, can never justify the deliberate killing of an innocent human being" (*EV*, n. 58, p. 105). This paragraph recapitulates many of the central claims of Pius XI in *CC*.

42. Ashley and O'Rourke, *Health Care Ethics*, 261, 253; Noonan, "Almost Absolute Value," 48–50; Connery, *Abortion*, 295–300. See discussion of principle of double effect in chapter 1.

43. Ashley and O'Rourke, *Health Care Ethics*, 253–54; Noonan, "Almost Absolute Value," 48; Connery, *Abortion*, 301–3; NCCB, "Ethical and Religious Directives for Catholic Health Care Services," n. 48, p. 458; John F. Tuohey, "The Implications of the 'Ethical and Religious Directives for Catholic Health Care Services' on the Clinical Practice of Resolving Ectopic Pregnancies," *Louvain Studies* 20 (1995): 41–57.

44. Grisez, *Abortion*, 340, and generally 333–41. Grisez (341–53) understands this argument to apply only for the purpose of saving the mother's life; preserving the mother's health, or any other good short of life, would not justify the death of the unborn child. Ashley and O'Rourke, *Health Care Ethics*, 261–62, appear to accept Grisez's view but do not explicitly endorse it.

45. Jakobovits, "Jewish Views on Abortion," 143, and generally 124–43.

46. Feinstein (who would allow abortion only if the threat to the mother's life were certain), *Iggerot Moshe* 7 Hoshen Mishpat 2, n. 69; Bleich, "Abortion in Halakhic Literature," 356; and others cited in Steinberg, *Encyclopedia of Jewish Medical Ethics*, vol. 2, 80–86. Issar Unterman, "On the Matter of Saving of the Life of a Fetus," *Noam* 6 (1963): 5, 1–11, considers abortion to be an appurtenance of murder, based partly on Rabbi Ishmael's midrashic reading of Genesis 9:6; because abortion is not fully considered murder, it is permitted when necessary to save life. Similarly Moshe Tendler writes that "abortion is tantamount to murder and can be sanctioned only when the life of the gestating mother is in danger" ("On the Interface of Religion and Medical Science: The Judeo-Biblical Perspective," in *Jewish and Catholic Bioethics: An Ecumenical Dialogue*, ed. Edmund D. Pellegrino and Alan I. Faden [Washington, D.C.: Georgetown University Press, 1999], 108). Abortion in such cases traditionally is justified by regarding the fetus as a *rodeif*, or (material) aggressor. Lisa Sowle Cahill observes, "Such analogies to assault serve simultaneously to protect the mother and the fetus. As David Novak illustrates by the Jewish comparison of a fetus to a 'pursuer,' references to a victim-aggressor conflict imply that the fetus is to be killed if and only if there exists the gravest reason, i.e., threat to the mother's life"; see "Abortion and Argument by Analogy," *Horizons* 9, no. 2 (1982): 277–78, citing David Novak, "Judaism and Contemporary Bioethics," *Journal of Medicine and Philosophy* 4 (1979): 357.

47. Bernard Häring, "A Theological Evaluation," in Noonan, *The Morality of Abortion*, 135, 138.

48. McCormick, "Public Policy on Abortion," 194–95.

49. Curran, "Abortion: Ethical Aspects," 222; "Abortion: Its Legal and Moral Aspects," 191.

50. Cahill, "Abortion, Autonomy, and Community," 86.

51. See Feldman, *Birth Control in Jewish Law*, 284–86; Bleich, "Abortion in Halakhic Literature," 362–63; Steinberg, *Encyclopedia of Jewish Medical Ethics*, vol. 2, 85.

52. Steinberg, *Encyclopedia of Jewish Medical Ethics*, vol. 2, 85–86; Bleich, "Abortion in Halakhic Literature," 354–56; Herring, *Jewish Ethics and Halakhah*, 40–42. Some thinkers, such as classical authority Joseph Trani,

understand the basic reason for the prohibition of abortion to be that it would represent impermissible self-injury for the woman. As the self-injury of amputation is allowed when it is required to improve health, so abortion would be permitted for this purpose.

53. Bokser and Abelson, "Statement on the Permissibility of Abortion," 195.

54. *Mishpetei Uziel* 3, *H.M.*, n. 46 (Jerusalem: Va'ad L'hotza'at Kitvei Harav, 1995), pp. 224, 221–26; and discussion in Feldman, *Birth Control in Jewish Law*, 289–91; Herring, *Jewish Ethics and Halakhah for Our Time*, 41; Bleich, "Abortion in Halakhic Literature," 355.

55. Feldman, *Birth Control in Jewish Law*, 290 (attributing this observation to Viktor Aptowitzer).

56. Daniel C. Maguire, "The Catholic Legacy and Abortion: A Debate," *Commonweal* 114 (1987): 678.

57. As reported by McCormick, "Notes on Moral Theology," 333, citing Bruno Ribes, "Dossier sur l'avortement: L'Apport de nos lecteurs," *Etudes* (April 1973), 511–34. An example of such an inhuman situation would be the birth of a child with such severe deformities as to preclude social relationships.

58. Christine Gudorf, "Making Distinctions," *Christianity and Crisis* 46 (1986): 242–44.

59. Waldenberg, *Tzitz Eliezer*, v. 13, n. 102, p. 209; v. 14, nn. 100–102, pp. 183–92. Waldenberg's concern with anguish and harming marital relationships parallels the views of Gudorf. In the extreme case of Tay-Sachs disease, Waldenberg presents, as a supplementary reason warranting abortion, concern to avoid suffering of the child in the future. Waldenberg emphasizes the need for seriousness and caution in all cases concerning abortion (v. 9, n. 51, sec. 3, p. 240; v. 14, n. 100, p. 186).

60. Kassel Abelson, "Prenatal Testing and Abortion," in Mackler, *Life and Death Responsibilities in Jewish Biomedical Ethics*, 219.

61. Solomon Freehof, "Abortion," in *American Reform Responsa*, ed. Walter Jacob (New York: Central Conference of American Rabbis, 1983), n. 171, p. 543.

62. Blu Greenberg, "Abortion: A Challenge to Halakhah," *Judaism* 25 (1976): 202–6.

63. Balfour Brickner, "Judaism and Abortion," in *Contemporary Jewish Ethics*, ed. Menachem Marc Kellner (New York: Sanhedrin, 1978), 287–88.

64. Ibid., 287; Balfour Brickner, "A Critique of Bleich on Abortion," *Sh'ma* 5, no. 85 (1975): 200.

65. "When Is Abortion Permitted?" in *Contemporary American Reform Responsa*, ed. Walter Jacob (New York: Central Conference of American Rab-

bis, 1987), n. 16, p. 27; Bokser and Abelson, "Statement on the Permissibility of Abortion," 195. Reform thinker Mark Washofsky writes, "Two broad conclusions emerge from this picture of a conversation between halakhic positions. The first is that a woman would not be entitled to abortion on demand; there must exist a warrant, a sufficient and carefully-reasoned justification for the procedure. The second is that the definition of 'sufficient' will differ from case to individual case" ("Abortion and the Halakhic Conversation: A Liberal Perspective," in *The Fetus and Fertility*, ed. Walter Jacob and Moshe Zemer [Pittsburgh: Rodef Shalom Press, 1995], 75). Although Conservative rabbi Robert Gordis supports abortion for compelling reasons and advocates generally permissive laws, he likewise condemns abortion on demand as immoral. "Abortion on demand is a threat to a basic ethical principle" of reverence for life. "When an embryo is aborted, we are, in the fine rabbinic phrase, 'diminishing the divine image in which man is fashioned'" ("Abortion: Major Wrong or Basic Right?" in Mackler, *Life and Death Responsibilities*, 228).

66. *EV*, nn. 58, 18; pp. 105, 30–31. See similarly "Declaration on Procured Abortion," n. 14, p. 446.

67. Ashley and O'Rourke, *Health Care Ethics*, 259. Ashley and O'Rourke insist that even in the most difficult circumstances, abortion is objectively wrong. "The right of the mother to compassion, however, is based on the same grounds as the child's right to life, so that human sympathy and justice must be given to both."

68. McCormick, "Notes on Moral Theology," 330. "One of the most important functions of morality is to provide to a culture the ongoing possibility of criticizing and transcending itself and its limitations. Thus genuine morality, while always compassionate and understanding in its meeting with individual distress (pastoral), must remain prophetic and demanding in the norms through which it invites to a better humanity (moral); for if it ceases to do this, it simply collapses the pastoral and the moral and in doing so ceases to be truly human, because it barters the good that will liberate and humanize for the compromise that will merely comfort" (ibid., 356). The bishops' statements McCormick is reviewing were issued in the early 1970s.

69. Häring, "Theological Evaluation," 141–42, quoting his *Shalom: Peace. The Sacrament of Reconciliation* (New York: Farrar, Straus, and Giroux, 1968). "Invincible ignorance should not be interpreted in the sense of mere intellectualism but rather in the light of a theory on conscience, which emphasizes the existential totality of man. Invincible ignorance is a matter of inability of a person to 'realize' a moral obligation. Because of the person's total experience, the psychological impasses, and the whole context of his life, he is unable to cope with a certain moral imperative" ("Theological Evalua-

tion," 140). As I have noted, Häring also suggests some leniency relative to magisterial views with regard to the morality of abortion.

70. Häring, "Theological Evaluation," 140, writes that "on the level of pastoral counselling a Catholic moralist might come to almost the same conclusion and even to almost the same way of friendly discourse as Gustafson." He refers here to James M. Gustafson's discussion of a case involving rape. Gustafson writes that he "could morally justify an abortion," "would affirm its moral propriety in this instance" to the woman, and would help provide resources to enable the woman to receive the abortion ("A Protestant Ethical Approach," in Noonan, *The Morality of Abortion*, 117–18). Gustafson notes possible affinities between his approach and that of some Catholics (120–21). McCormick, "Notes on Moral Theology," 339–42, suggests that what Gustafson refers to as moral justification might better be termed pastoral justification. Regardless of whether Gustafson would agree, McCormick's construal may well reflect Häring's understanding of the position with which he is expressing significant agreement.

71. McCormick, "Notes on Moral Theology," 330.

72. *EV*, n. 59, pp. 105–6.

73. "Declaration on Procured Abortion," nn. 23, 26, pp. 449–50.

74. Häring, "Theological Evaluation," 144.

75. Lisa Sowle Cahill, "Abortion, Sex, and Gender: The Church's Public Voice," *America* 168, no. 18 (1993): 7–8.

76. Maguire, "Catholic Legacy and Abortion," 661–62.

77. Jakobovits, "Jewish Views on Abortion,"142, 139.

78. Greenberg, "Abortion: A Challenge to Halakhah," 204–7. See also Gordis, "Abortion: Major Wrong or Basic Right?" 228–29.

79. Cahill, "Abortion, Sex, and Gender," 7. She claims that "relative to the rest of the culture, American Catholics are fighting one another for turf on a number of 'hot' issues . . . all within about three notches of the right end of a spectrum reaching from one to ten."

80. Häring, "Theological Evaluation," 132. Häring refers to "milder opinions which were proposed by renowned Catholic moralists," although over the last century "the Holy See has more and more eliminated" these opinions.

81. Ashley and O'Rourke, *Health Care Ethics*, 256, note this agreement, though they frame the consensus somewhat more conservatively: "Disagreement on how to deal with rare conflict cases does not negate the basic agreement among Jews and all the Christian churches (1) that abortion is contrary to the will of God, who creates each human person, and (2) that if abortion is ever permissible in a conflict situation . . . it can be justified only by the most serious reasons. This ought to be a basis for religious Jews, Protestants,

Orthodox, and Catholics to work together to decrease the great number of abortions in our country."

82. "Respect for Life: Jewish and Roman Catholic Reflections on Abortion and Related Issues," Board of Rabbis of Southern California Interfaith Committee, Los Angeles Chapter of the American Jewish Committee Interreligious Affairs Committee, and Roman Catholic Archdiocese of Los Angeles Commission on Ecumenical and Interreligious Affairs, Los Angeles: September 1977.

83. Richard A. McCormick cites Paul Ramsey's observation that "far more than any argument, it was surely the power of the nativity stories and their place in ritual and celebration and song that tempered the conscience of the West to its audacious effort to wipe out the practice of abortion and infanticide" (Richard McCormick, *Health and Medicine in the Catholic Tradition* [New York: Crossroad, 1987], 53, quoting Paul Ramsey, "Liturgy and Ethics," *Journal of Religious Ethics* 7 [1979]: 139–71). See also *EV*, n. 45, p. 80.

84. Häring complains, "In the past, contraception and abortion were somehow put on the same or equal level: as a crime against nature and against the procreative function of sexuality. . . . The encyclical *Casti connubii* is probably the most classical official text that condemns contraception and abortion with almost the same severe expressions" ("Theological Evaluation," 133–34). For Sanchez the prohibition against contraception is more stringent than that against abortion (see note 8). Pope Sixtus V, in the bull *Effraenatam*, imposed the penalties of homicide both on abortion—at any stage of gestation—and on contraception (Noonan, "Almost Absolute Value," 33). As I have noted, rabbis Yair Bachrach and Jacob Emden understood abortion to violate the prohibition against contraception. For Jewish thinkers, see also Steinberg, *Encyclopedia of Jewish Medical Ethics*, vol. 2, 77; Feldman, *Birth Control in Jewish Law*, 251–53.

85. See Feldman, *Birth Control in Jewish Law*; John T. Noonan, *Contraception: A History of Its Treatment by the Catholic Theologians and Canonists*, rev. ed. (Cambridge, Mass.: Belknap Press, Harvard University Press, 1986). A full evaluation of the reasons for differences regarding contraception is beyond the scope of this book. One difference appears to be the greater normative importance of biological teleology in Catholic thought. In addition, Judaism consistently has understood sexual relations between husband and wife to be positive and indeed a mitzvah, or religious obligation. Although normative Catholicism has accepted and appreciated marital sexual relations, significant Catholic sources have portrayed sex as inherently sinful (at least in the current world, after the fall) or justified only by procreative intent. In Judaism, marriage is normative and abstinence from sex is gener-

ally disfavored. In Catholicism, celibacy represents a component of "the more perfect way" of religious life. John Paul II writes that although marriage should be esteemed, "the church throughout her history has always defended the superiority of this charism [celibacy] to that of marriage, by reason of the wholly singular link which it has with the kingdom of God" (*Familiaris Consortio: On the Family* [Washington, D.C.: United States Catholic Conference, 1982], n. 16, p. 14). Accordingly, the option of a married woman simply abstaining from sexual relations when pregnancy would endanger her health better coheres with the Catholic tradition than with the Jewish tradition. See also Pius XII, "The Apostolate of the Midwife," in *The Major Addresses of Pope Pius XII*, ed. Vincent A. Yzermans (St. Paul, Minn.: North Central Publishing Co., 1961), vol. 1, 170.

86. See similarly the observation of Cardinal Joseph Bernadin, *The Consistent Ethic of Life* (Kansas City, Mo.: Sheed and Ward, 1988), 58: "The consistent ethic of life is primarily a theological concept, derived from biblical and ecclesial tradition about the sacredness of human life, about our responsibilities to protect, defend, nurture and enhance God's gift of life."

Chapter 6

In Vitro Fertilization

Both Judaism and Roman Catholicism value the family and understand the full blessings of marriage to include children as well as loving companionship. For both traditions, marriage and sexual relations include unitive and procreative dimensions. Procreation normatively occurs within marriage, and—at least in the ideal case—conception arises from marital intercourse.

Complications arise when a married couple wishes to have children but is not able to do so. Infertility has been a concern throughout human history. The Bible reports that women such as Sarah, Rebecca, and Hannah suffered because of their infertility. Rachel cried to her husband Jacob, "Give me children, or I shall die."[1] About 7 percent of couples in the United States are infertile—unable to have children after one year or more of trying to do so. A variety of medical and technological interventions have been developed, which help many infertile couples to have a child.[2] Religious thinkers have raised questions about which of these interventions are morally appropriate. For Jewish and Catholic writers alike, having children represents an area in which medicine must be practiced in a manner consistent with responsible and reverent stewardship. Differences arise with regard to how to specify and balance values such as human dignity, love of neighbor, compassion, healing, and a human stewardship that is both active and respectful of divine sovereignty.

One of the most dramatic interventions is in vitro fertilization (IVF). IVF involves fertilization of an ovum outside the body; "in vitro," literally meaning "in glass," refers to the laboratory equipment in which sperm and ova are combined. In the first successful use of IVF as a reproductive technology, British researchers Robert Edwards and Patrick Steptoe fertilized an ovum produced by Leslie

Brown with sperm produced by her husband and transferred the fertilized ovum to her uterus, leading to the birth of Louise Brown in July 1978. As the technique typically is practiced today, a woman preparing for IVF receives hormones to stimulate development of several ova. Shortly before ovulation would occur, a physician uses ultrasound to guide a needle through the cervix to the ovaries to gather developed ova, which are combined with prepared sperm. One or more resulting embryos are allowed to develop for a period of up to a few days, reaching the stage of two to eight cells, and are then transferred to a woman's uterus for implantation and gestation. At the two- to eight-cell stage, embryos also could be cryopreserved or "frozen" for transfer at a later time. IVF originally was developed to assist women with damaged or absent fallopian tubes. The fallopian tube, connecting the ovary and uterus, typically is the site of fertilization as well as the path by which the fertilized ovum reaches the uterus. IVF also has been used in response to other female infertility factors, such as endometriosis or ovulatory problems; for male infertility factors; and for "unexplained infertility."[3]

Opposition to In Vitro Fertilization

The Roman Catholic magisterium and many Catholic theologians—as well as a few Jewish authorities—oppose all use of IVF, including homologous cases in which a husband's sperm and wife's egg give rise to an embryo that is implanted in the wife for gestation.[4] Catholic opponents of IVF tend to focus on three related concerns. Most generally, IVF represents an inappropriate approach of domination to procreation. Second, it severs the link between marital intercourse and having children. Finally, such procedures are unjust to the child who is born; they subject the child to the risk of injury and foster an attitude of treating the child as a product. Several additional concerns also have been expressed. As commonly practiced, IVF involves the death of embryos that are in excess of the number the couple wishes to implant. Sperm usually is obtained by masturbation, which generally is prohibited by both Catholic and Jewish tradition. There is a risk of gametes or in vitro embryos being mixed up, leading inadvertently to a heterologous case (using gametes from outside the marriage). For many IVF opponents, even if these ancillary concerns could be addressed IVF would remain wrong.

All of these concerns are joined in *Donum Vitae*, the Vatican Congregation for the Doctrine of the Faith's "Instruction on Respect for Human Life in Its Origin and on the Dignity of Procreation: Replies to Certain Questions of the Day." Although *Donum Vitae* strongly condemns heterologous IVF, it devotes greater attention to explaining its rejection of homologous cases as well. A central concern is that IVF, like contraception, is incompatible with the inseparable connection between the unitive and procreative meanings of marital intercourse. As with contraception, linking unitive and procreative aspects within a couple's overall relationship is not sufficient because individual actions must be judged in themselves. "Homologous artificial fertilization, in seeking a procreation which is not the fruit of a specific act of conjugal union, objectively effects an analogous [to contraception] separation between the goods and the meanings of marriage." The common use of masturbation to obtain sperm for IVF is a "sign" of the wrongful dissociation of unitive and procreative in IVF generally. Marital relations normatively express the couple's mutual self-gift and openness to new life. "Fertilization achieved outside the bodies of the couple remains by this very fact deprived of the meanings and the values which are expressed in the language of the body and in the union of human persons." Such procreation would be "deprived of its proper perfection." The couple's natural desire for a child, their suffering, and the possibility of subjectively admirable intentions are acknowledged, but these factors cannot justify that which is intrinsically wrong.[5]

Artificial procreation intrinsically fails to respect the dignity of the child born from such procedures. "The one conceived must be the fruit of his parents' love. He cannot be desired or conceived as the product of an intervention of medical and biological techniques; that would be equivalent to reducing him to an object of scientific technology."[6] *Donum Vitae* expresses concerns for in vitro embryos as well. "From the moment the zygote has formed, [it] demands the unconditional respect that is morally due to the human being in his bodily and spiritual totality." *Donum Vitae* not only condemns the destruction of human embryos, it also asserts that manipulation of embryos fails to respect their dignity and cryopreservation exposes them to unacceptable risks. Although the destruction of embryos is anathema, the essential problems of IVF are those involving sex and procreation. "The Church remain[s] opposed from the moral point of view to homologous 'in vitro' fertilization. Such fertilization is in itself illicit and in opposition to the dignity of procreation and of the conjugal union, even when everything is done to avoid the death of the human embryo."[7]

Opposition to the wrongful domination of procreation provides a theme that runs throughout *Donum Vitae*, linking the aforementioned concerns. "In the conjugal act . . . the spouses cooperate as servants and *not as masters* in the work of the Creator who is Love." The introduction to *Donum Vitae* begins by noting that although some therapeutic interventions to assist with procreation are licit, new procedures enable some people "to *dominate* the process of procreation," exceeding man's "reasonable dominion." When in vitro embryos are selected for implantation, "the researcher usurps the place of God; and, even though he may be unaware of this, he sets himself up as the *master* of the destiny of others inasmuch as he arbitrarily chooses whom he will allow to live and whom he will send to death. . . . Through these procedures, with apparently contrary purposes, life and death are subjected to the decision of man, who thus sets himself up as the giver of life and death by decree. This dynamic of violence and *domination* may remain unnoticed by those very individuals who, in wishing to utilize the procedure, become subject to it themselves. . . . The abortion-mentality which has made this procedure possible thus leads, whether one wants it or not, to man's *domination* over the life and death of his fellow human beings." In addition to concern for embryos is that for children born of these procedures. "No one may subject the coming of a child into the world to conditions of technical efficiency which are to be evaluated according to standards of *control and dominion*." In sum:

> Homologous IVF and ET [embryo transfer] is brought about outside the bodies of the couple through actions of third parties whose competence and technical activity determine the success of the procedure. Such fertilization entrusts the life and identity of the embryo into the power of doctors and biologists and establishes the *domination* of technology over the origin and destiny of the human person. Such a relationship of *domination* is in itself contrary to the dignity and equality that must be common to parents and children.[8]

Donum Vitae's rejection of reproductive technologies continues the views of Pope Pius XII. Pius briefly addressed IVF—while it was still being developed—in his 1956 address to the Second World Congress on Fertility and Sterility. "On the subject of the experiments in artificial fecundation '*in vitro*,' let it suffice Us to observe that they must be rejected as immoral and absolutely illicit." In this speech he referred to an earlier (1949) address in which he rejected both heterologous and (somewhat less vehemently) homologous artificial insemination. "We must never forget this: It is only the procreation of a new life according to the will and plan of the Creator which brings with it—to an astonishing degree of perfection—the realization of the desired ends. This is, at the same time, in harmony with the dignity of the marriage partners, with their bodily and spiritual nature, and with the normal and happy development of the child." In a 1951 allocution, Pius elaborates on the requirement for procreation to take place only following "the conjugal act," which expresses the mutual self-giving and union of the couple. "This is much more than the mere union of two life-germs." "To reduce the cohabitation of married persons and the conjugal act to a mere organic function for the transmission of the germ of life would be to convert the domestic hearth, sanctuary of the family, into nothing more than a biological laboratory."[9]

Elio Sgreccia emphasizes concerns with domination in recapitulating central themes of *Donum Vitae*, including the connection between disrespect for human sexuality and disrespect for human persons. IVF represents the attempt to "dominate the procedures of human procreation. . . . Artificial procreation presents itself as a severing of the link of obedience between procreators and creator; it implies the refusal of God's transcendent design." Furthermore, it represents "man's domination over man, which is contrary to respect for life as God's gift and a transcendent value. . . . Only if conception is the fruit of human love and not of deterministic technique, will the human being enter history supported by love and free from biotechnological influence." Reproductive technologies represent "the technical act which builds the object," in which "the subject who built the object can dominate it"; this approach to procreation contrasts with "the act which expresses the subject to another subject, whose equality he respects," through which procreation appropriately occurs.[10]

William E. May and Joseph Boyle also present themselves as summarizing the major arguments of *Donum Vitae*; however, they emphasize the inconsistency of IVF with respect for children born of the procedures. May asserts that "it is morally wrong to choose to generate human life outside the marital act"—defined as an act of intercourse between husband and wife that is both "(1) open to the communication of spousal love and (2) open to the reception of new human life." "When human life is given through the marital act it comes, even when ardently desired, as a 'gift' crowning the act itself. The marital act is not an act of 'making.'"[11] With IVF, however, the child is made as a product; the child "comes in existence, not as a gift supervening on an act expressive of the marital union . . . but rather in the manner of a product of a making (and, typically, as the end product of a process managed and carried out by persons other than his parents)."[12] Such an act of conscious production to meet parental desires demeans the child. "A choice to bring about conception in this fashion inevitably means willing the baby's initial status as a product. But this status is subpersonal, and so the choice to produce a baby is inevitably the choice to enter into a relationship with the baby, not as an equal, but as a product inferior to its producers." There is an unacceptable risk that parents will reject a child who appears to them to be defective. Even if the parents eventually develop an appropriate relationship of care for the child, however, that result would not justify the initial violation of respect for human dignity.[13]

Joseph Boyle, Jr., argues similarly that respect for the child is the keystone of *Donum Vitae*'s argument. The inseparability of unitive and procreative meanings when a marital act occurs does not necessarily imply that one may not procreate in the absence of a marital act; the "Instruction" extends the inseparability principle precisely because procreation outside the marital act fails to respect the child. "In reproductive activities which do not meet its condition, the child in its coming-to-be is treated as an object, a thing and not a person. The sign and the fruit of mutual self-giving are not products made, but are a gift and blessing welcomed. By contrast, the results of productive activities cannot but be regarded as things having a status inferior to those who make them."[14] Ashley and O'Rourke add that "it is unjust to children to bring them into the world without the assurance that they originated in the natural marital act of their parents," expressive of the parents' union, because doing so would weaken the child's security and its bond to its parents.[15]

Cardinal Joseph Bernadin presents *Donum Vitae* in a more moderate tone, often raising questions for the reader's consideration rather than asserting definitive conclusions. Cardinal Bernadin expects wide agreement with two central principles: "the inviolable dignity of every human life," including embryos, and "the essential and necessary relationship between human sexuality, marriage and parenthood"—ruling out donor gametes. Bernadin acknowledges that a third principle is more controversial: Like marriage itself, "the act of intercourse which celebrates and incarnates the meaning of marriage also has two purposes: lovemaking and life making. And just as these aspects cannot be separated in marriage, so too they cannot be separated in marital intercourse." Bernadin suggests that the creation of life may be qualitatively different from other activities and that reproductive technology may be "tampering with something so fundamentally human that we are endangering the quality of future life." A practice of homologous IVF could expand to more problematic applications and make "possible an attitude which would encourage a couple genetically planning a 'perfect' child to resist or reject anything less than their ideal."[16]

Jewish thinkers overwhelmingly accept IVF, at least in homologous cases and with appropriate safeguards. Some Orthodox Jewish authorities, however—including Rabbi Eliezer Yehudah Waldenberg—oppose IVF even in homologous cases. Waldenberg frames his concerns not in terms of the intrinsic nature of sex but in terms of specific halakhic prohibitions. Although he accepts artificial insemination in exceptional cases, with IVF scientists have more extended control over gametes and embryos, so there is a higher risk of confusion. This situation could lead to problems entailed by donor gametes, including the risk of consanguinity as children sharing an unknown biological parent come to marry. The procurement and manipulation of sperm for IVF violates the traditional prohibition of "emission of seed in vain," *hotza'at zera l'vattalah*.[17] The violation is more blatant than it is for artificial insemination because in IVF most sperm remains outside the woman's reproductive tract.[18]

Waldenberg argues that IVF cannot be considered as, and does not facilitate, natural reproduction. IVF "upsets the order of creation." It is impossible to view the husband or wife as truly a parent of the off-spring because not they but a "third power" causes both fertilization and implantation. The husband would not fulfill the traditional mitzvah to "be fruitful and multiply" (*p'ru ur'vu*, Genesis 1:28—which is understood to require that a couple give birth to at least one girl and one boy).[19] Like Sgreccia and others, Waldenberg warns that the practice of IVF will expand. IVF will lead to cloning and to a "test tube child" who is conceived and gestated extracorporeally, with no human connection. Truly human procreation will be lost, leading to chaos and complexities reaching "to the highest heavens." Therefore IVF must be absolutely forbidden.[20]

In Vitro Fertilization in Homologous Cases

Three general themes dominate arguments for the legitimacy of IVF, at least in homologous cases. One theme is that intervening in nature to facilitate procreation is morally and theologically acceptable. It is natural for humans to use reason and technology in responding to challenges, as evidenced by the practice of medicine. Such active intervention can be an appropriate expression of active human stewardship. A second theme—of greatest concern to Catholic authors—addresses the connections among procreation, marriage, and sex. In this line of argument, unitive and procreative aspects are joined in the actions and intentions of the couple, especially when the overall context of the couple's marriage is considered. Even if procreation ideally follows marital intercourse, when that is not possible IVF and other uses of reproductive technologies are legitimate. A third general theme emphasizes that a couple's desire for a biological child is legitimate. Infertility often engenders suffering, and a child born with the help of IVF can add to the joy and fulfillment of the family. In addition to these three major themes, various authors address several additional concerns, including the treatment of embryos and the procurement of sperm.

Richard McCormick briefly addresses these ancillary questions. The very early embryo, which has not yet individualized, deserves a measure of respect but not equal to that accorded persons; IVF could be acceptable despite the fact that it entails some deaths of early embryos.[21] Masturbation to produce sperm for procreative purposes is acceptable because it represents "a different human action" than masturbation for pleasure, which he condemns.[22]

McCormick's major focus, however, is *Donum Vitae*'s claims regarding the inseparability of unitive and procreative aspects. He expresses general agreement with this principle but criticizes the magisterium for applying it in too rigid a way—focusing narrowly on individual acts and biological faculties rather than on the person "integrally and adequately considered." McCormick suggests that "it might be sufficient if the spheres of the unitive and procreative are held together so that there is no procreation apart from marriage, and no full sexual intimacy apart from a context of responsibility for procreation." Inseparability is "to be realized in the relationship, not in the individual acts."[23] In this context, the procreative intervention of IVF can be unitive, in expressing and strengthening the couple's unitive bond. The procedures of IVF can represent acts of love and indeed may be seen as extensions of the couple's sexual intimacy. McCormick grants that ideally unitive and procreative aspects are combined in every act, for aesthetic reasons if no others, but this ideal is not an absolute requirement. "All artificial interventions . . . are a kind of 'second best,'" entailing disvalues, so conception through IVF is "deprived of its proper perfection," as *Donum Vitae* asserts. "However, a procedure 'deprived of its proper perfection' is not necessarily morally wrong in all cases."[24]

Like McCormick, Lisa Sowle Cahill appeals to a criterion of "the human person integrally and adequately considered" and argues that the connection of unitive and procreative should be considered in the context of the couple's overall relationship. "The one inviolable value in the marital-sexual-parental scenario would be the love union of the couple, understood to extend to their domestic, social, and parental relationship." IVF may be regarded as "an assisted fulfillment" of the couple's sexual intimacy. *Donum Vitae* articulates an appropriate ideal for marital sexuality and procreation, but Cahill questions whether "the terms of the evaluations allow for sufficient sensitivity to situations in which the attainment of a reasonably defined ideal is obstructed by practical circumstances? What might such sensitivity require in the cases at hand?" When a couple is not able to have a child through sexual intercourse, homologous IVF is appropriate. "Homologous methods permit a couple to retain the constitutive physical relationship of marriage, i.e., sexual intercourse, the constitutive physical relationship of parenthood, i.e., genetic reproduction, and the physical relationship which unites spousehood and parenthood, i.e., a mutual genetic contribution to offspring."[25]

Cahill addresses briefly additional issues, including the value of adoption as an alternative to reproductive technologies, the extent to which reproductive technologies should represent a priority for society, and the danger that women especially will feel inappropriate pressure to use these means.[26] She considers at greater length the treatment of embryos. The in vitro embryo "has very considerable value and makes very significant claims, but it is not the equivalent of a 'baby.'" It is reasonable to accept some loss of embryos as inevitable because natural fertilization leads to significant loss.[27] At the same time, "there is a moral obligation to minimize embryo loss, even if as a consequence the chance of pregnancy will not be optimal."[28]

Sidney Callahan expresses views akin to those of McCormick and Cahill, but she focuses on the acceptability of artificial intervention in procreation rather than on the connection of unitive and procreative. "An ethic based solely on the natural biological integrity of marital acts will not serve, because the mastery of nature through technological problem solving is also completely natural to us—indeed, it is the glory of *homo sapiens*." Simply accepting a "technological imperative" and catering to individuals' desires, however, risks harm to children, families, and society as a whole. Callahan proposes an "ethical standard of medical remediation and restoration of a married couple's average expectable fertility" and argues that this standard supports homologous IVF.[29]

John Mahoney argues similarly against attacks on IVF as unnatural. He criticizes a static mindset that assumes that because in the past there was only one way to achieve a goal, such as procreation, that way is now the only legitimate approach. "The characteristically human qualities are intelligent control of the environment coupled with respect, and simple human ingenuity in finding means to ends. In more religious terms, the difference is one between the passive acceptance of God's gifts and finding in them the challenge of active stewardship."[30] The use of technology does not preclude marital union and loving acts as the basis for procreation. The procedures of IVF can be a couple's "expression of deep mutual love and of a shared longing to give each other a child as the fruit of their married life and love. . . . And if science can now bring to birth this living expression of the love between husband and wife which would otherwise simply not exist, this too, it would appear, must be seen as part of the Creator's loving plan for all his children."[31] Mahoney also argues that obtaining sperm by masturbation is acceptable. Masturbation generally is condemned because of its "biological futility and emotional futility. But neither of these considerations is applicable in the cases which we have been considering, where the production of semen is directed towards reproduction and is a physical expression of marital and parental love." In general, Mahoney argues, homologous IVF for a married couple is acceptable.[32]

Jewish writers overwhelmingly accept IVF, at least in appropriate homologous cases. They generally point to considerations similar to those raised by Catholic thinkers, though with less attention to issues of unitive and procreative dimensions of sex. Jewish writers are more likely to express positive views toward IVF, judging it not only acceptable but commendable because it represents an appropriate therapeutic intervention that enables the couple to have a child. One group of authors explicitly distinguish their understanding from that of *Donum Vitae*. "Like the Roman Catholic *Instruction*, *halakhah* considers natural marital procedures to be morally normative; but it does not regard them to be morally absolute. . . . Accordingly, the religious obligation to procreate can sometimes outweigh the imperative to maintain natural procedures and homologous artificial insemination or in vitro fertilization (IVF) might be allowed to overcome a fertility problem." The authors note that Genesis 1:28 combines calls both to be fruitful and multiply and to exercise dominion over nature. Controlling nature in a morally responsible way can represent the fulfillment of God's will.[33]

Orthodox rabbi J. David Bleich similarly asserts that Judaism does not accept the Catholic Church's natural law arguments against IVF and contraception. "In the absence of a specific prohibition, man is free to utilize scientific knowledge to overcome impediments of nature." Bleich rejects Waldenberg's claims regarding the artificial character of IVF and sees a clear distinction between "capricious genetic manipulation" and "in vitro fertilization which simulates natural procreation and is designed solely to alleviate infertility." Bleich does express concern for in vitro embryos, understanding them to be included in a strict prohibition against abortion. Accordingly, he recommends fertilization of only one ovum for transfer. Bleich also worries about the risk of defects in children born of IVF. "It will require the birth and maturation through adolescence and into adulthood of a significant number of healthy and normal test-tube babies before the technique may be viewed as morally acceptable." Nevertheless, Bleich offers a positive if qualified endorsement of IVF. "If properly controlled . . . this revolutionary technology can be a welcome means of bestowing the happiness and fulfillment of parenthood upon otherwise childless couples."[34]

Other Orthodox authorities express a permissive stance toward discarding in vitro embryos that have not been designated for transfer to a womb and are unwanted.[35] General support for IVF is offered by Orthodox rabbi Avigdor Nebenzal, who writes in response to Waldenberg's prohibition. Prohibiting IVF, even as a last resort, could prevent fulfillment of the traditional mandate of procreation. It could increase the couple's anguish, bitterness of spirit, and psychological suffering. On a more technical point, producing sperm to fertilize an egg would not represent "emission of seed in vain" because the husband's intention is procreative. For Nebenzal, IVF differs only superficially from natural procreation. Although IVF raises some legitimate concerns, these concerns may be outweighed by consideration of the happiness of the couple in the community of Israel.[36]

Conservative rabbi David Feldman offers similar considerations in support of IVF. IVF need not be rejected as unnatural. "The process of creation is ongoing, and we seek to be 'partners with God' in conquering and controlling nature. . . . Hence, giving nature a little help when, for example, Fallopian tubes are blocked, by circumventing this impediment through use of the Petri dish, is quite acceptable, even meritorious." Moreover, the couple's desire for a child is appropriate and should be supported. "The desire of a woman for offspring is a deeply human one, and helping her realize this desire is a positively human deed. As long as we can safeguard against abuse, it is a mitzvah to resort, if necessary, to laboratory assistance to help bring about this desired end." In sum, "with so pronatalist a general and specific tradition, the Jewish response has been understandably affirmative to new reproductive techniques, such as in-vitro fertilization."[37]

Similar views are expressed in a responsum approved by the Conservative movement's Committee on Jewish Law and Standards.[38] Optimally, children should be conceived through marital sexual relations when possible.[39] When required, however, "medical interventions to assist the natural process of reproduction" could be appropriate and compatible with "our responsibility to be both reverent and active in our partnership with God." Possible risks to children born from IVF and women undergoing the procedures must be considered, but experience shows these risks to be not prohibitive in most cases. The procedures entail significant burdens on couples (especially women), so IVF is not obligatory.[40] Nevertheless, "it is clear that IVF is permissible for those who choose to utilize these procedures. For these couples, technical and other halakhic concerns are outweighed by the great good of a new human life, the addition to the harmony and joy of the family, and the contribution to the strengthening of the Jewish community and humanity. A child born as a result of IVF using a couple's sperm and egg is fully the parents' child in all respects, and causes the mitzvah of 'be fruitful and multiply' to be fulfilled."[41]

The Conservative responsum allows the creation of more than one embryo at a time, to improve the likelihood of success and minimize the burdens on the woman of repeated egg retrievals. "The early embryo should be accorded a significant degree of respect and sanctity as a wondrous divine creation and potential human life." Nevertheless, the early in vitro embryo has a somewhat lower status than in utero fetus. The former has not reached the stage of individualization, and because of its location it is not on a natural trajectory of development. Although embryos that the couple does not want to implant could be kept frozen indefinitely or donated, discarding in vitro embryos in the context of IVF procedures would not be prohibited.[42]

Similar arguments are made in a responsum from the Reform movement. IVF is supported as a form of "healing, a medical response to the disease of infertility." Moreover, IVF can enable Jews to fulfill the mitzvah of procreation. "The positive value of IVF as a medical therapy clearly justifies the necessary discarding of embryos" because the in vitro embryo is not a person (though it should be respected as a "person 'in becoming'").[43] Another Reform writer supports IVF as expanding "procreative autonomy"—a crucial though not absolute value.[44]

Opposition to Donor Gametes

Many thinkers who accept IVF in homologous cases reject the use of donor gametes. Some writers have argued that such use is intrinsically wrong and is likely to harm both individuals involved and society more broadly. The use of donor gametes radically separates marriage and procreation and violates marital exclusivity. It confuses the child's genealogy, threatening the child's sense of identity and weakening the relation of parent and child. The donor contributes to the birth of a child without assuming responsibility to care for the child, separating biological and personal aspects and encouraging sexual irresponsibility in society. Heterologous IVF defers too strongly to individual choice and fosters attitudes of eugenics and viewing children as products.

Thinkers who oppose all IVF generally condemn heterologous uses as especially offensive. For *Donum Vitae*, heterologous IVF violates the unity of marriage and mutual responsibilities of husband and wife. It destroys the natural link of marriage, biological parenthood, and care for the child. The use of donor gametes violates the right of the child because it "deprives him of his filial relationship with his parental origins and can hinder the maturing of his personal identity." This disconnect harms relationships within the family and (more subtly) society in general.[45] Cardinal Bernadin similarly condemns the use of donor gametes, which violates the widely recognized "essential unity between marital sexual intimacy and the generation of new life."[46] For Jewish opponents of IVF such as Waldenberg, one of the most powerful objections to homologous IVF is the risk of confusion of gametes or embryos, leading to inadvertent heterologous cases, with confusion of genealogy and the risk of consanguineous marriage.[47]

Many writers who accept homologous IVF reject heterologous usage. Such rejection is the dominant stance of Catholic writers, who frequently argue that whereas homologous IVF retains the unity between procreation and marriage, the use of donor gametes violates this connection. For example, Richard McCormick states that "conjugal exclusivity should include the genetic, gestational, and rearing dimensions of parenthood. Separating these dimensions . . . too easily contains a subtle diminishment of some aspect of the human person." As I have noted, McCormick regards IVF as an extension of the couple's sexual intimacy; from this perspective, the involvement of a third person who contributes gametes is especially intrusive. The use of donor gametes also introduces a harmful asymmetry in the relation of parents to the child. "It brings into the world a child with no bond of origin to one or both marital partners, thus blurring the child's genealogy and potentially compromising the child's self-identity." By radically separating procreation from marriage, heterologous IVF is likely to encourage unmarried individuals to have children and to increase adultery. It would distort the family and basic values by exaggerating the importance of childbearing, as well as encouraging eugenics and a "stud-farm mentality."[48]

Lisa Sowle Cahill also sharply distinguishes between homologous and heterologous IVF. The former maintains the unity of love, sex, marriage, and parenting, in the context of the couple's relationship if not in each individual act. The latter breaks this unity, harming or failing to respect all involved. A married couple must forgo donor gametes to "testify that their unity as spouses is more important than realizing the physical reproductive potential of one without the other, that there is a natural unity of the intentional and physical dimensions of spousehood and parenthood which should not be broken deliberately." The use of donor gametes violates the spouses' "commitment to marital cooperation and fidelity." An imbalance is introduced into the relationship of both parents to the child, and "the child's 'natural' relation of offspring to parent is impaired." Heterologous methods also are inappropriate vis-à-vis the donor, whose biological and reproductive capacities are alienated from the donor's life as a person. In general, heterologous methods overemphasize choice and treat family relationships as matters of contract, instead of respecting the givenness of embodied human life and natural ties.[49]

Sidney Callahan articulates similar concerns in arguing for IVF only in homologous cases. The use of donor gametes violates the couple's "marital and biological unity." "The intruding third-party donor, as in adultery, will inevitably have a psychological effect on the couple's life. Even if there is no jealousy or envy, the reproductive inadequacy of one partner has been made definite, and reliance has been placed on an outsider's potency, genetic heritage, and superior reproductive capacity." Psychology and sociobiology indicate the importance of shared genes and biological connections in supporting family relationships of love and care; when biological links are absent, problems tend to become exacerbated if the family comes under stress. Most troubling are the risks for children born from heterologous interventions. The child would be estranged from its genetic lineage and biological relatives. The child will resent parents "who have had it made to order" and the donor who was not "concerned with what would happen to the new life he or she helped to create." "Treating the child like a commodity—something to be created for the pleasure of the parents infringes upon the child's dignity." Callahan expresses views similar to those in *Donum Vitae* in insisting on natural procreation (which she construes, however, to include homologous IVF). "When one is begotten (not made), then one shares equally with one's parents in the ongoing transmission of the gift of life from generation to generation. The child procreated in the expectable way is a subsidiary gift arising from the prior marital relationship, not a product or project of the parental will." Heterologous reproduction will harm society by weakening the family and trivializing sexuality and reproduction.[50]

Within Judaism, Orthodox thinkers generally oppose the use of donor gametes, for many of the same reasons offered by Catholic writers.[51] For example, Bleich—though accepting homologous IVF in principle—insists that "such procedures can, of course, be sanctioned only if the sperm of the husband is used exclusively."[52] Bleich elaborates his concerns in discussing artificial insemination. A married woman's use of another man's sperm might be considered adultery and is minimally "a repugnant violation of the marital relationship." Concealment of genealogy is inherently problematic and could lead to consanguineous marriage among biological siblings.[53]

Perhaps most forceful in attacking the use of donor gametes is Orthodox rabbi Immanuel Jakobovits, who expresses concerns similar to those of Catholic opponents of artificial technologies—often using similar language. For example, Jakobovits opposes donor insemination "without reservation as utterly evil." It "severs the link between the procreation of children and marriage, indispensable to the maintenance of the family as the most basic and sacred unit of human society." Similarly, he condemns IVF with donor gametes:

> Man, as the delicately balanced fusion of body, mind and soul, can never be the mere product of laboratory conditions and scientific

ingenuity. To fulfill his destiny as a creative creature in the image of his Creator, he must be generated and reared out of the intimate love joining husband and wife together, out of identifiable parents who care for the development of their offspring, and out of a home which provides affectionate warmth and compassion.[54]

Acceptance of Donor Gametes

Some theologians acknowledge many of the foregoing concerns but accept the use of donor gametes in appropriate cases. They may concede that heterologous IVF deviates from the ideal more severely than does homologous IVF, that couples should reflect carefully before proceeding with such actions, and that couples who use donor gametes must consider how to deal with the real problems entailed. Nevertheless, the use of donor gametes could be consistent with, and in fact express, marital love and commitment. The child—who otherwise would not have existed—may be brought up with love and support. Individuals may donate gametes with a sense of responsibility and altruism. Although the problems of donor gametes mandate caution, they do not rule out the procedure in all cases.

Perhaps most notably among Catholic theologians, Louis Janssens has argued for the acceptability of donor sperm in the context of artificial insemination. Donor insemination is acceptable only when husband and wife acknowledge (and do not try to hide) their infertility, are committed to caring for the child, and "if both have the necessary qualities for psychological parenthood." The child could receive a "normal upbringing," as do adopted children, and likely would not resent the choice of the couple. "Will it cause a shock for the child if the parents explain that AID [donor insemination] was chosen (for eugenic reasons) to protect the child against the risk of a serious hereditary defect?" The donor's actions could be appropriate if (for example) he and his wife decide to help another couple experience the joy of having children; they could determine that "the giving of sperm . . . does not harm their mutual love but, on the contrary, enriches them by proving their conscious yet disinterested service to another couple in need." Although donor insemination entails negative aspects, these factors may be outweighed in some cases.

With responsible selection, the positive aspects of the experience of those involved in AID supersede the lack of complete biological parenthood. . . . The couple who seek AID do not see it as a personal act of infidelity to each other or as a threat to their love relationship. On the contrary, many experience the help for their childlessness as so enriching for their relationship as a couple that a growing number request it to conceive a second and sometimes a third child.[55]

Paul Lauritzen emphasizes personal and relational considerations. He agrees with thinkers such as Cahill that human relationships are embodied but claims that this embodiment may occur in the physical interactions of spouses and of parents and children, not only through biology and genetics. "A child may be the embodiment of a couple's love and care in a sense that is every bit as real as the embodiment of their love in the physical sense that he is flesh of their flesh."[56] Having a child through heterologous methods does not deny the bodily nature of humans. "Caring for children—however they are conceived—is no mere assertion of the will but is a bodily affair from start to finish. DI [donor insemination] no more challenges the meaning of embodiment than does any other effort to overcome physical (embodied) obstacles," such as the use of prosthetic limbs. Parents legitimately may have a child using donor gametes only when they commit themselves irrevocably and unconditionally to love and care for the child, as do adopting parents. Common practices such as secrecy supported by lies and denial of the donor's significance are harmful but need not be followed. The gamete donor should be recognized as a real person, and some information should be made available to the child about his or her genetic parent. The asymmetry of the child's relationship to mother and father poses real challenges, but this admitted element of "disunity" need not be an "overwhelming obstacle to responsible parenthood." Asymmetries and potential conflicts are successfully negotiated in many blended families, and the potential for conflict exists with all children and families. "The potential strains of asymmetry may be mediated by an honest, loving, and straightforward acknowledgment of the differences between families created through the use of donor gametes and those created 'naturally.'" "If we value the rearing function of parenthood more highly than the genetic relation of biological parenthood, and if we assess the forms of pursuing parenthood in relation to the standards of responsible parenthood so understood, donor insemination cannot be categorically rejected, even if it can be advocated only cautiously." Although Lauritzen focuses on donor insemination, he notes that his arguments apply as well to the use of donor gametes in IVF. Indeed, the asymmetry involved with donor eggs is less pronounced than that with donor sperm because the woman experiences the biological relationship of gestation and birth.[57]

Lauritzen's distinction between egg and sperm donation is found in a more pronounced form among some Jewish thinkers. In traditional halakhah, the man who contributes sperm is recognized as the child's natural father. In cases of egg donation, both the woman who donates the egg and the woman who gestates and gives birth to the child have biological connections to the child. For most Jewish authorities, gestation and birth are the primary determinants of maternity. Accordingly, when donor sperm is utilized by a couple, the husband in effect adopts the son of another man. When donor eggs are used, and the wife gestates and gives birth to the child, she may be regarded as a natural mother.

Orthodox authorities especially express greater concern with sperm donation than with egg donation and discuss the legitimacy of this practice in greater depth.[58] Although Orthodox authorities generally oppose the use of donor gametes (especially sperm), some allow their use—cautiously and on a case-by-case basis—to allow the birth of a child and to relieve suffering of a particular couple who cannot be reconciled to childlessness or adoption. Responding to a request by a couple for permission to use donor sperm, Moshe Feinstein writes, "One may permit in very pressing circumstances, when they are suffering greatly in their longing for a child."[59]

Conservative and Reform theologians accept and expand this approval. Like Janssens and Lauritzen, they acknowledge the concerns raised by opponents of donor gametes as significant but not necessarily decisive. The use of donor gametes does not constitute adultery or violate any intrinsic prohibition. In some cases the negative aspects of heterologous IVF would be outweighed by positive values of giving birth to new life and enabling the couple to have a child, relieving their suffering and strengthening their family. Within the Conservative movement, a groundbreaking work on accepting donor gametes was a responsum by Rabbi Elliot Dorff on donor insemination. For Dorff, technical concerns raised by some Orthodox rabbis are not decisive: Donor insemination does not constitute adultery or violate marital fidelity, and unintentional incest is very unlikely, especially if records are maintained and relevant information made available to children and their families. Dorff quotes Lauritzen in noting that personal challenges to the couple and family (including those of asymmetry) are profound but can be addressed effectively. Given the lack of compelling considerations forbidding donor insemination, compassion mandates support for couples choosing to use heterologous procedures (as well as affirmation of couples' choices not to use such procedures). This support is reinforced by the tradition's emphasis on the value of procreation and communal demographic concerns in the wake of the Holocaust.[60]

Dorff writes that a man may donate sperm, but only with a thoughtful appreciation of the responsibilities entailed. "He should approach this whole process . . . with a sense of mitzvah, duly appreciative of the awesomeness of the human ability to procreate and of his role in helping that happen for an infertile couple." The donor should make information regarding physical and personal characteristics available to the child, although the donor may retain anonymity with regard to specific identifying information. Similar concerns would apply to a woman donating eggs, although she also would need to consider the medical risks involved.[61]

The Conservative responsum on IVF concurs with and expands Dorff's position, accepting in appropriate cases the use of donor gametes or embryos. "Couples considering the use of donated sperm, ova, or embryos should consider the halakhic and personal concerns involved, should receive thorough counseling, and should seriously investigate alternatives, including adoption. Those wishing to use donated sperm, ova, or embryos may do so." Similarly, "after careful consideration of the implications of their actions, a couple may donate an embryo formed from their sperm and egg to enable another couple to have a child."[62]

Reform Jewish writers tend to accept the use of donor gametes— often with less hesitancy than their Conservative colleagues. Rabbi Solomon Freehof writes that because donor insemination does not constitute adultery and the likelihood of consanguineous marriage is remote, the procedure should be permitted. Rabbi Alexander Guttman responds that there is cause for discomfort with such procedures; they need not be prohibited, but they should not receive an unqualified endorsement. Rabbi Walter Jacob offers "reluctant permission" for a couple to use an egg donated by a first cousin in IVF; because the donor is known, there is concern that the cousin may be unduly pressured to donate, and other "psychological difficulties" may ensue.[63] David Ellenson cautiously supports donor insemination and heterologous IVF, adding that children should have some right to information regarding "their biological origins."[64] A recent Reform responsum states that although the genetic parents are the child's natural parents, a couple using donor gametes simply become the child's parents by adoption. Unlike other writings I have surveyed, this responsum notes no psychological or other concerns that need be addressed by couples using heterologous procedures, or in evaluating this practice generally.[65]

Conclusion

In addressing in vitro fertilization—as with other issues—Jewish and Christian writers generally express similar views. Each tradition articulates a norm of procreation occurring within marriage, ideally as a result of sexual intercourse. IVF and other uses of reproductive technologies are evaluated in relation to this ideal and within a broader understanding of appropriate human stewardship. Attention also is given to the well-being of children born of such procedures, their families, and society more broadly.

Within each tradition, some thinkers condemn all use of IVF as incompatible with appropriate human procreation. Others respond that such human intervention into natural processes of procreation can be consistent with ethical values and responsible stewardship. Thinkers in both traditions recognize that the use of donor gametes entails special concerns. Some condemn all heterologous procedures as intrusive on the relationship of husband and wife and harmful to children born of the procedures and their relationship with parents. Others argue that the problems of donor gametes can be dealt with in a way that would allow their use in appropriate cases.

Jewish and Catholic judgments regarding IVF represent overlapping spectra of acceptance. The range of Jewish views tends to be more accepting of such procedures in general and of the use of donor gametes in particular. The considerations raised by writers in the faith communities also generally overlap, although they diverge in some ways. Catholic writers attach greater importance to the inseparable connection between marital sexual relations and procreation. For the magisterium and others, this connection prohibits any IVF. Even Catholics who accept IVF generally grant that the inseparability is absolute, though they argue that this requirement may be met within the broader context of a marriage rather than in each individual act. Relatively few Catholic writers are willing to accept the use of donor gametes, though a few argue that such actions may express marital love without violating sexual fidelity. For most Jewish writers, the connection of marital sex and procreation represents an ideal that should be maintained when possible. When interventions are required for a couple to have a child, however, these interventions may be accepted. Even the few Jewish writers who reject all IVF do not appeal to an absolute need to connect sex and procreation.[66]

More generally, some Catholics oppose IVF as contravening God's plan as manifested by biology and nature. IVF constitutes a wrongful attempt to dominate nature, rather than more passively remaining open to procreation. Other Catholics respond that although natural procreation may represent the ideal, when that ideal outcome cannot occur medical interventions can be appropriate and consistent with God's will. Jewish writers address this issue and overwhelmingly support such beneficial interventions in the natural order, developing arguments similar to those of their Catholic counterparts. Jewish writers are more likely to commend human intervention as an example of humans acting as partners with God. Precedents for this understanding may be found in the Talmud, which speaks of three partners in the creation of a human being, each offering vital contributions: the mother, the father, and God.[67]

A difference between the traditions, familiar from chapter 5, concerns in vitro embryos. For the magisterium and other Catholic opponents of IVF, the likely death of such embryos, or even the risks entailed by IVF procedures, represent an absolute bar to IVF because the embryos must be respected as persons. Although this is not the central argument presented against IVF, this consideration likely strengthens the opposition of the magisterium and others. Some Catholic writers accept IVF that involves some risk to embryos, though they may insist on restrictions to minimize this risk, in part because in vitro embryos do not have the full status of personhood. There also is a common appeal to the general biology of human functioning, of the sort often associated with more conservative theologians: When a couple engages in sexual intercourse, many embryos naturally fail to implant and therefore become discarded. Although most Jewish writers call for a degree of respect for the in vitro embryo, none regard it as a person or prohibit all IVF on this basis. Most accept the death of in vitro embryos within the context of IVF; most would accept the death of some embryos to minimize burdens on the woman or increase the chances of success.[68] This position is justified by the imperative of healing, generally without appeals to natural biological activity.

Catholic writers are much more likely than Jewish writers to worry that IVF demeans and harms the child. The magisterium and others assert that IVF is intrinsically wrong and inherently treats the child as a product, manufactured as a means to fulfill desires, rather than as a person equal to the parents. Other Catholics accept homologous IVF as an appropriate extension of natural reproduction but claim that the use of donor gametes inherently treats the child as a product made to fulfill parental wishes and therefore must be rejected. Although some Jewish authors reject all IVF, and many reject the use of donor gametes, none do so on the basis that such procedures unacceptably fail to respect the child.[69] Concern is expressed to assure the medical safety of the procedures. Jewish and Catholic authors who accept the use of IVF, or the use of donor gametes, urge the importance of parents manifesting appropriate attitudes of love and care.

Jewish authors tend to emphasize the positive warrants in favor of IVF, presenting IVF as not only acceptable but welcome. They portray infertility as a disease and include the use of reproductive technologies within in the paradigm of healing. Moreover, most Jewish writers understand the birth of a child through IVF to represent fulfillment of the mitzvah of "be fruitful and multiply," at least in homologous cases.[70] Although such artificial interventions are not considered obligatory, they are encouraged for couples who choose to utilize them in appropriate cases.

Jewish writers more consistently affirm the positive value of a couple having a child using IVF. They are more likely than Catholic authors to accept the use of IVF to avoid the couple's suffering. In a review article, Edward Vacek argues that for the magisterium and some Catholic theologians, suffering is regarded as "a morally extrinsic consideration, to be handled as a spiritual theme, but not part of the moral reckoning itself."[71] For most Jewish writers, suffering is very much part of the reckoning. The decisive role of this consideration is clearest in the discussion of donor gametes.[72] Compassion and a commitment to avoid the couple's suffering leads some Orthodox authorities to accept the use of donor gametes in exceptional cases, despite these authorities' objections to and distaste for such interventions. For Conservative rabbi Elliot Dorff, compassion provides a decisive value supporting his approval of donor gametes in appropriate cases.[73]

In general, Jewish and Catholic writers express similar concerns in their discussion of IVF, and the two faith communities exhibit overlapping ranges of views with regard to the acceptability of IVF (both homologous and heterologous). Within this broad picture, Catholic authors tend to give more weight to natural biological functioning, as well as to protection of embryos. Jewish authors tend to take an activist stance toward the use of reproductive technologies, supported by values of healing, procreation, and compassion.[74]

Notes

1. Genesis 16–18, 25; I Samuel 1; Genesis 30:1. The Bible relates that God was mindful of each of these women, and each gave birth to a child. Men's infertility is described less commonly; polygamy was practiced in biblical times, and Isaac, Jacob, and Elkanah had children with other wives. Abraham speaks of his being childless in praying to God (Genesis 15:3).

2. New York State Task Force on Life and the Law, *Assisted Reproductive Technologies: Analysis and Recommendations for Public Policy* (New York: New York State Task Force on Life and the Law, 1998), 10–13.

3. Canadian Royal Commission on New Reproductive Technologies, *Proceed with Care: Final Report of the Royal Commission on New Reproductive Technologies* (Ottawa: Royal Commission on New Reproductive Technologies, 1993); American Fertility Society, Ethics Committee, "Ethical Considerations of Assisted Reproductive Technologies," *Fertility and Sterility* 62 (November 1994, suppl.): 35S—36S; New York State Task Force, *Assisted Reproductive Technologies*, 51–60. I use the term "embryo" broadly in this

chapter to refer to the product of fertilization throughout its early development. Because of the rudimentary nature of its development at this stage, some prefer the term "preembryo" (American Fertility Society) or "zygote" (Canada). See also the discussion of the status of the fetus in chapter 5.

4. This chapter addresses the use of IVF only by a married couple that seeks to have offspring. Virtually no Jewish or Catholic writers endorse the use of IVF by unmarried individuals. Moreover, although some unmarried women wish to use donated sperm to reproduce, relatively few seek (or require) IVF procedures.

5. Congregation for the Doctrine of Faith, *Donum Vitae: Instruction on Respect for Human Life in Its Origin and on the Dignity of Procreation: Replies to Certain Questions of the Day [DV]* (Washington, D.C.: United States Catholic Conference, 1987), II.B.4–8, pp. 26–34.

6. Ibid., II.B.4, p. 28.

7. Ibid., I (pp. 12–20); II: Introduction (p. 21), B.5 (p. 31).

8. Ibid., II.B.4 (p. 28), Introduction (p. 5), I.5 (p. 18), II: Introduction (pp. 21–22), II.B.5 (p. 30); emphasis added.

9. "Marriage and Parenthood," *The Pope Speaks* 3 (1956): 194; "Address to the 4th International Convention of Catholic Physicians," in *Readings in Moral Theology, no. 8: Dialogue about Catholic Sexual Teaching*, ed. Charles E. Curran and Richard A. McCormick (Mahwah, N.J.: Paulist, 1993), 223–24; "Discourse on Moral Problems of Married Life," in ibid., 225.

10. Elio Sgreccia, "Moral Theology and Artificial Procreation in Light of *Donum Vitae*," in *Gift of Life: Catholic Scholars Respond to the Vatican Instruction*, ed. Edmund D. Pellegrino, John Collins Harvey, and John P. Langan (Washington, D.C.: Georgetown University Press, 1990), 116, 126–28, 132. Reproductive technologies contribute to a project of "anthropotechnics," in which humans manufacture and manipulate other humans. This project recalls J. Robert Oppenheimer's reported assessment of the development of the atom bomb: "We are working for the devil" (116).

11. William E. May, "Catholic Teaching on the Laboratory Generation of Human Life," in *The Gift of Life: The Proceedings of a National Conference on the Vatican Instruction on Reproductive Ethics and Technology*, ed. Marilyn Wallace and Thomas W. Hilgers (Omaha, Neb.: Pope Paul VI Institute Press, 1990), 89, 82–84. May's argument in this work is similar to that found in his "*Donum Vitae*: Catholic Teaching Concerning Homologous *In Vitro* Fertilization," in *Infertility: A Crossroad of Faith, Medicine and Technology*, ed. Kevin Wm. Wildes (Dordrecht, Netherlands: Kluwer, 1997), 73–92.

12. May, "Catholic Teaching," 84–85, quoting Catholic Bishops Committee on Bioethical Issues, *In Vitro Fertilization: Morality and Public Policy* (London: Catholic Information Services, 1983), n. 24.

13. May, "Catholic Teaching," 85. Jean Porter notes differences in the emphases and arguments of May and *Donum Vitae*, despite May's citation of the "Instruction" and agreement in rejecting IVF. According to *Donum Vitae*, unitive and procreative meanings are naturally joined in the sexual act, and the central problem of IVF "is its intrusiveness at the very point of conception." Violation of the dignity of the child follows from violation of the inseparability principle. For May, the central concern is respect for persons, understood in Kantian terms. Porter argues that May "grounds the moral meanings of human sexuality in free, self-determining choice" rather than in its natural characteristics. See Jean Porter, "Human Need and Natural Law," in Wildes, *Infertility*, 99–102.

14. Joseph Boyle, Jr., "An Overview of the Vatican's Instruction on Reproductive Ethics," in Pellegrino, Harvey, and Langan, *The Gift of Life*, 24–25. Boyle also objects that in IVF embryos are harmed, but he emphasizes that rejection of IVF does not depend on this concern.

15. Benedict M. Ashley and Kevin D. O'Rourke, *Health Care Ethics: A Theological Analysis*, 4th ed. (Washington, D.C.: Georgetown University Press, 1997), 246. The authors also condemn masturbation regardless of purpose (241).

16. Joseph Bernadin, "Science and the Creation of Life," *Origins* 17 (1987): 24–25.

17. The emission of sperm is especially problematic because Waldenberg does not recognize the husband as the father of a child born from IVF. On the concept of emission of seed in vain—also termed "destruction of seed" (*hashhatat zera*)—see David M. Feldman, *Birth Control in Jewish Law*, rev. ed. (Northvale, N.J.: Jason Aronson, 1998), 109–31. The term generally applies to masturbation, which some Orthodox authorities prohibit in all cases. Other Orthodox authorities express a strong preference for other means of procuring semen (ideally by obtaining it from the vagina following intercourse, otherwise by coitus interruptus or use of a condom) but allow masturbation when necessary for fertility testing and some forms of artificial reproduction. Indeed, Waldenberg himself allows masturbation in some cases as a last resort when it is required for fertility testing—asking that the man maintain pure thoughts during the procedure, intent on the mitzvah of procreation. See *Tzitz Eliezer*, 2d ed. (Jerusalem: n.p., 1985), vol. 9, n. 51, p. 207; Yoel Jakobovits, "Male Infertility: Halakhic Issues in Investigation and Management," *Tradition* 27, 2 (1993): 4–21.

18. Waldenberg, *Tzitz Eliezer*, vol. 15, n. 45, pp. 115–20.

19. The fourteenth-century *Sefer Hahinnukh* of Rabbi Aaron Halevy of Barcelona traces the mitzvah to Gen. 1:28, though other halakhic sources link the commandment to God's communication with Noah (Gen. 9:1, 7) or Jacob

(Gen. 35:11). Mishnah *Yevamot* 6:6 states, "One must not abstain from 'fruit-fulness and increase' unless one has children. The School of Shammai say: two males. The School of Hillel say: a male and a female, as it is written, 'male and female He created them' [Gen. 1:27]." Traditional Jewish law follows Hillel's view but encourages one to continue to engage in procreation even if one already has a son and a daughter—representing an additional mitzvah of *lashevet*, to inhabit the world, derived from Isaiah 45:18. Although having children (specifically, a boy and a girl) represents the fulfillment of a mitzvah, those who are unable to have children are exempt from the obligation. Indeed, J. David Bleich, *Judaism and Healing* (New York: Ktav, 1981), 113, argues that the mitzvah of procreation is best understood not as having children, which is beyond one's control, but as continuing one's practice of potentially procreative intercourse with one's spouse at least until a boy and a girl are born. Traditional Jewish law describes the obligation to procreate as incumbent upon males. This formulation (exegetically based on the wording of Gen. 1:28) may reflect a sociological background in which men have greater control than women over whether they would marry and procreate or a view that women should be encouraged but not technically obligated to undergo the risks of pregnancy and childbirth. See Joseph Karo, *Shulḥan Arukh*, *Even Ha'ezer* 1; David M. Feldman, *Health and Medicine in the Jewish Tradition* (New York: Crossroad, 1986), 69–71; idem, *Birth Control in Jewish Law*, 46–59; Elliot N. Dorff, "Artificial Insemination: General Considerations and Insemination Using the Husband's Sperm," in *Life and Death Responsibilities in Jewish Biomedical Ethics*, ed. Aaron L. Mackler (New York: Jewish Theological Seminary of America, Finkelstein Institute, 2000), 18–20, 30–32.

20. Waldenberg, *Tzitz Eliezer*, vol. 15, 118–19. Moshe Sternbuch also opposes IVF, sharing many of Waldenberg's objections. In IVF the test tube represents a separate power that is responsible for fertilization, so the husband would not truly be father to the child and would not fulfill the mitzvah of procreation. Accordingly, emission of sperm for use in IVF would be prohibited. The likelihood of confusion among gametes and embryos risks consanguinity and future disaster (Moshe Sternbuch, "Test-Tube Baby," *Bishvilei Harefu'ah* 8 [5747/1987]: 29–36). See also Avraham Steinberg, *Encyclopedia of Jewish Medical Ethics* (Jerusalem: Schlesinger Institute, 1988), s.v. "In Vitro Fertilization," 2: 129.

21. Richard McCormick, "Therapy or Tampering? The Ethics of Reproductive Technology and the Development of Doctrine," in *The Critical Calling: Reflections on Moral Dilemmas since Vatican II* (Washington, D.C.: Georgetown University Press, 1989), 343–46. See similarly Bernard Häring, *Medical Ethics*, ed. Gabrielle L. Jean (Notre Dame, Ind.: Fides, 1973), 93, and the discussion in chapter 5 on the status of early embryos.

22. McCormick, "Therapy or Tampering?" 337. See similarly Häring, *Medical Ethics,* 92–93, and the acceptance of "medically indicated masturbation" in Anthony Kosnik et al., *Human Sexuality: New Directions in American Catholic Thought* (New York: Paulist, 1977), 227.

23. McCormick, "Therapy or Tampering?" 338–40, 346–47. Häring, *Medical Ethics,* 92, earlier expressed a similar understanding regarding artificial insemination with the husband's sperm. "When the sperm comes from the husband and the whole marriage is lived in a climate of love, then not only is he biologically the father but there is not that total severance between the unitive and the procreative meaning of marriage." Alternatively, McCormick (337) suggests the possibility of narrowly construing "the inseparability of the unitive and procreative in the conjugal act." "If the conjugal act is performed, these dimensions may not be separated," but this "implies nothing about artificial reproduction beyond the marital act." (As I have noted, Boyle mentions but rejects such an interpretation.)

24. McCormick, "Therapy or Tampering?" 348–49. See similarly Edward V. Vacek's claim: "The typical logic of the Vatican's sexual ethics, it seems to me, is to state the ideal and then to insist that anything willfully short of the ideal is sinful. It slides from 'best way' to 'only way'" ("Notes on Moral Theology: Vatican Instruction on Reproductive Technology," *Theological Studies* 49 [1988]: 129).

25. Lisa Sowle Cahill, *Sex, Gender, and Christian Ethics* (Cambridge: Cambridge University Press, 1996), 238, 231–32; idem, "Moral Traditions, Ethical Language, and Reproductive Technologies," *Journal of Medicine and Philosophy* 14 (1989). 516.

26. Cahill, *Sex, Gender, and Christian Ethics*, 243–49; idem, "*In Vitro* Fertilization: Ethical Issues in Judaeo-Christian Perspective," *Loyola Law Review* 32 (1986): 344–46. Maura A. Ryan explores these issues in *Ethics and Economics of Assisted Reproduction: The Cost of Longing* (Washington, D.C.: Georgetown University Press, 2001). Ryan generally shares Cahill's cautious acceptance of assisted reproduction, at least some cases (51–56).

27. Vacek suggests that this natural loss argues against attributing the status of personhood to early embryos. "If every conceptus is a person, then in regularly engaging in sexual intercourse a fertile couple do an action that normally will lead to the death of a number of innocent persons each year" ("Notes on Moral Theology," 122). Louis Janssens, though generally affirmative in his evaluation of reproductive technologies, expresses concern about the death of embryos, although he does not reject IVF on this basis. "Even in the natural conception of human life a significant number of fertilized ova will be lost as a type of natural selection. But does that fact itself justify a consciously chosen manner of acting? Can this satisfy the moral demand to protect human life with

the greatest of care from the moment of its conception?" ("Artificial Insemination: Ethical Considerations," Louvain Studies 7 [1980]: 25).

28. Cahill, "In Vitro Fertilization," 348–54. Cahill also considers the consequences of IVF for particular families and for society more broadly; although consequences are not necessarily decisive, they support the use of IVF in appropriate homologous cases (344–47).

29. Sidney Callahan, "The Ethical Challenge of the New Reproductive Technology," in Health Care Ethics: Critical Issues for the 21st Century, ed. John F. Monagle and David C. Thomasma (Gaithersburg, Md.: Aspen, 1998), 46–47.

30. John Mahoney, Bioethics and Belief: Religion and Medicine in Dialogue (London: Sheed and Ward, 1984), 15–16. See similarly the argument of Janssens, "Artificial Insemination," 20: "What is one to do in those cases in which the natural efficiency, so strongly emphasized by Hürth (une téléologie presque incroyable), of sexual intercourse to conceive new life breaks down and is in fact inefficient? Is it not obvious in such cases to appeal to reason, that is also part of human nature, to investigate how to alleviate such factually present inefficiency?"

31. Mahoney, Bioethics and Belief, 15–17.

32. Ibid., 14–15, 30. Mahoney also notes concerns with decisions to leave embryos unimplanted and with treating embryos as commodities, but these concerns do not preclude the appropriate use of IVF (ibid., 30–32).

33. Richard V. Grazi, Joel B. Wolowelsky, and Raphael Jewelewicz, "Assisted Reproduction in Contemporary Jewish Law and Ethics," Gynecological and Obstetric Investigations 37 (1994): 218. Wolowelsky is an Orthodox rabbi; Grazi and Jewelewicz are physicians. They cite the writings of Rabbi Joseph Soloveitchik: "Only the man who builds hospitals, discovers therapeutic techniques, and saves lives is blessed with dignity. . . . Man reaching for the distant stars is acting in harmony with his nature, which was created, willed, and directed by his Maker. It is a manifestation of obedience to rather than rebellion against God" ("The Lonely Man of Faith," Tradition 7 [1965]: 5–67). See also Steinberg, Encyclopedia of Jewish Medical Ethics, 2: 124–29.

34. Bleich, Judaism and Healing, 86–91; idem, Contemporary Halakhic Problems IV (New York: Ktav and Yeshiva University Press, 1995), 238–42. Bleich raises the possibility that abortion restrictions may not apply to an early in vitro embryo because of the embryo's microscopic size, so embryos could be discarded (Bioethical Dilemmas: A Jewish Perspective [Hoboken, N.J.: Ktav, 1998], 209–11).

35. Hayyim David Halevi, "On Fetal Reduction and the Halakhic Status of In Vitro Embryos," Assia, no. 47–48 (1990): 14–17; Mordechai

Eliyahu, "Destroying Fertilized Eggs and Fetal Reduction," *Teḥumin* 11 (1991): 272–74.

36. Avigdor Nebenzal, "In Vitro Fertilization: Notes," *Assia*, no. 35 (1983): 5. Nebenzal's acceptance of the use of the husband's sperm parallels the views of McCormick and others.

37. Feldman, *Health and Medicine*, 71–72.

38. Aaron L. Mackler, "In Vitro Fertilization," in Mackler, *Life and Death Responsibilities*, 97–122. The endorsement of the Rabbinical Assembly's Committee on Jewish Law and Standards reflects authorization beyond my individual views.

39. Mackler refers to the medieval *Iggeret Hakodesh*: "The union of man with his wife, when it is proper, is the mystery of the foundation of the world and its civilization. Through the act they become partners with God in the act of creation. This is the mystery of what the sages said, 'When a man unites with his wife in holiness, the *Shekhinah* [divine presence] is between them in the mystery of man and woman'" ("In Vitro Fertilization," 115); *The Holy Letter*, trans. Seymour J. Cohen (Northvale, N.J.: Jason Aronson, 1993; reprint of New York: Ktav, 1976), 92.

40. "As expressed by Rabbi Elliot Dorff, 'The Jewish tradition would have all people, fertile or infertile, understand that our ability to procreate is not the source of our ultimate, divine worth; that comes from being created in God's image.' Individuals who cannot have children can make other vital contributions to strengthening the Jewish (and human) community" (Mackler, "In Vitro Fertilization," 102, quoting Dorff, "Artificial Insemination: The Use of a Donor's Sperm," in Mackler, *Life and Death Responsibilities*, 38).

41. Mackler, "In Vitro Fertilization," 101–2.

42. Ibid., 105–12.

43. Central Conference of American Rabbis, "In Vitro Fertilization and the Status of the Embryo," www.ccarnet.org/cgi-bin/respdisp.pl?file= 2&year=5757. Discarding of embryos is considered necessary because many embryos must be created for IVF procedures to be effective, and preserving every embryo would impose unrealistic burdens on facilities.

44. David Ellenson, "Artificial Fertilization (*Hafrayyah Melakhotit*) and Procreative Autonomy: In Light of Two Contemporary Israeli Responsa," in *The Fetus and Fertility: Essays and Responsa*, ed. Walter Jacob and Moshe Zemer (Pittsburgh: Rodef Shalom Press, 1995), 33.

45. *Donum Vitae*, II.A.2, pp. 24–25. "Heterologous artificial fertilization is contrary to the unity of marriage, to the dignity of the spouses, to the vocation proper to parents, and to the child's right to be conceived and brought into the world in marriage and from marriage" (24). The Instruction cites Pope Pius

XII's 1949 "Address to the 4th International Convention of Catholic Physicians," which raises similar objections (see above). In turn, *Donum Vitae* is cited by Ashley and O'Rourke, *Health Care Ethics*, 245, among others.

46. Bernadin, "Science and the Creation of Life," 24.

47. See Waldenberg, *Tzitz Eliezer*, vol. 15, 116, 119, and discussion above.

48. McCormick, "Therapy or Tampering?" 330, 341–43. Häring, *Medical Ethics*, 92, likewise criticizes the use of donor gametes because of "the total separation of procreation from the unitive aspect of sexuality." John Mahoney, *Bioethics and Belief*, 34, 18–23, expresses "reservations" about the use of donor gametes, based "on the nature of marriage and family as understood by belief." He does not find to be persuasive arguments based on negative consequences anticipated from heterologous procedures. Mahoney more strongly opposes attitudes that a person has a "right to have a child," and procreation by unmarried persons.

49. Cahill, "Moral Traditions," 516–20; idem, "*In Vitro* Fertilization," 347–48; idem, *Sex, Gender, and Christian Ethics*, 232–33. "It is wrong in the process of formulating moral norms to take human biology and dissociate it from total personal existence. To treat a donor as an anonymous nonpersonal provider of a commodity which can be introduced into two of the most crucial and most intimate relationships of other persons, marriage and parenthood, is to do just that" (Cahill, "In Vitro Fertilization," 348). Cahill does offer support for embryo donation to protect in vitro embryos (and, implicitly, because some of the problems of gamete donation would not apply). With technological developments such as cryopreservation of embryos, "it is more likely that every healthy embryo can have the opportunity for implantation and thus a chance of survival, either in its genetic mother or by adoption. . . . A strict obligation to reimplant all embryos in optimal settings would involve soliciting adoptive wombs, . . . [manifesting] a strong view of the status of the early embryo" (Cahill, "In Vitro Fertilization," 354).

50. Callahan, "Ethical Challenge," 49–54.

51. See Steinberg, *Encyclopedia of Jewish Medical Ethics*, vol. 2, 129–30; Grazi et al., 222–24.

52. Bleich, *Judaism and Healing*, 89. Bleich adds for emphasis, "Under no circumstances should the sperm of any person other than the husband be utilized."

53. Ibid., 82–83. Bleich may be especially troubled by sperm donation because he—like most other authorities—considers the provider of sperm to be recognized as the child's father in halakhah. Maternity is determined primarily by gestation and birth, however, so the woman who gestates an embryo that is donated or arises from a donated egg is recognized as the child's natural mother.

The child is reared by its mother, so problems of genealogy are obviated. See Bleich, *Contemporary Halakhic Problems IV*, 237–72, and discussion below.

54. Immanuel Jakobovits, *Jewish Medical Ethics*, rev. ed. (New York: Bloch, 1975) 248–49, 266, citing *AJA Review*, London (spring 1974) 13–14. This argument parallels the language of Pope Pius XII's 1951 address: "To reduce the cohabitation of married persons and the conjugal act to a mere organic function for the transmission of the germ of life would be to convert the domestic hearth, sanctuary of the family, into nothing more than a biological laboratory" ("Discourse on Moral Problems of Married Life," October 29, 1951, in *Readings in Moral Theology*, 225). Like McCormick and others, Jakobovits depicts donor insemination as stud farming (*Jewish Medical Ethics*, 248).

55. Janssens, "Artificial Insemination," 25–29. Janssens continues: "Obviously these rather positive experiences must be critically considered in the light of the personalist criterion: the person adequately considered in himself and in his relations. They have certainly converged to such an extent that in my humble opinion morality can no longer speak in terms of complete condemnation, rather it must emphasize that this is a delicate matter in which very circumspect selection both of the couple and of the donor is demanded" (29).

56. Paul Lauritzen, "Pursuing Parenthood: Reflections on Donor Insemination," *Second Opinion* 17, no. 1 (1991): 61. Lauritzen writes of his own experience with donor insemination: The "desire to have a child of our 'own' was not a desire for genetic offspring; it was a desire for our union in a child. And if we could not have a child that was the result of our physical union, we could have a child that was the product of our spiritual union, who might also happen to have Lisa's smile" (58).

57. Ibid., 61, 72, 75, and 57–75 generally; Paul Lauritzen, *Pursuing Parenthood: Ethical Issues in Assisted Reproduction* (Bloomington: University of Indiana Press, 1993), 96–97. Vacek, "Notes on Moral Theology," 115, 125–26, raises similar considerations. Heterologous reproduction could involve loving marital acts and "agapic affirmation of a spouse's fertility." Although the use of donor gametes will lead to a "distorted family," in some cases that situation may be preferable to a family with no child.

58. Although adoption has become recognized increasingly over the centuries, de facto and for many purposes de jure, natural parents are still traditionally regarded as determinative for some purposes of Jewish law—such as whether a child receives synagogue honors as a *kohein* (a descendant of the biblical *kohanim*, or priestly clan). On the determination of parentage and its significance, see Steinberg, *Encyclopedia of Jewish Medical Ethics*, vol. 2, s.v. "In Vitro Fertilization," 129–38, and vol. 1, s.v. "Artificial Insemination," 154–59; Bleich, *Contemporary Halakhic Problems IV*, 237–72; Aaron L.

Mackler, "Maternal Identity and the Religious Status of Children Born to a Surrogate Mother," in Mackler, *Life and Death Responsibilities*, 174–87; Dorff, "Artificial Insemination: Donor's Sperm," 42–49; idem, "Artificial Insemination: Using Donor Eggs, Donating Sperm and Eggs, and Adoption," in Mackler, *Life and Death Responsibilities*, 84–87.

59. Moshe Feinstein, *Iggerot Moshe* (Brooklyn, N.Y.: Moriah, 1961), *Even Ha'ezer* 1, no. 71, p. 170. See Richard V. Grazi and Joel B. Wolowelsky, "Donor Gametes for Assisted Reproduction in Contemporary Jewish Law and Ethics," *Assisted Reproductive Reviews* 2 (1992): 157–60. Although Shlomo Auerbach expresses greater reluctance, he agrees that donor insemination is not absolutely prohibited. Despite his distaste for the procedure, he recognizes that for some couples who wish to use donor sperm, "this is truly a question of life" ("Artificial Insemination," *Noam* 1 [1958]: 159, 165–66). Both Feinstein and Auerbach specify that the donor should not be Jewish, arguing that a Jewish biological father would involve greater concerns regarding lineage and potential consanguinity.

60. Dorff, "Artificial Insemination: Donor's Sperm," 37–74.

61. Dorff, "Artificial Insemination: Donor Eggs," 82, and 81–84, 88–89 generally.

62. Mackler, "In Vitro Fertilization," 112–13; similarly 107–8.

63. *American Reform Responsa*, ed. Walter Jacob (New York: Central Conference of American Rabbis, 1983) 500–505; *Contemporary American Reform Responsa*, ed. Walter Jacob (New York: Central Conference of American Rabbis, 1987), 31–32.

64. Ellenson, "Artificial Fertilization (*Hafrayyah Melakhotit*) and Procreative Autonomy," 34–36. Ellenson endorses Maura Ryan's call for attention to social and relational considerations and cites her as stating that heterologous IVF "would be acceptable 'as the risks to the donor are small and the benefit great'" (34, citing Maura A. Ryan, "The Argument for Unlimited Procreative Liberty: A Feminist Critique," *Hastings Center Report* 20, no. 4 [1990]: 11).

65. Central Conference of American Rabbis, "In Vitro Fertilization." "In the event that a child is born to or raised by parents other than those who donated the sperm and the egg, he or she becomes the adoptive child of those parents. This does not present inordinate difficulties under Jewish law. . . . The child adopted by another couple has no legal or religious relationship to the donors of the egg and sperm, although for personal, medical, and genetic reasons the child or his/her guardian should be permitted to discover the identity of the biological parents at an appropriate time."

Noam J. Zohar, an Orthodox academic, finds in Feinstein's acceptance of donor gametes and some authorities' denial of paternity for a child born from artificial insemination "the kernel of a more radical proposal." Individual choice, together with human acts of parenting, may determine the child's parents. Zohar suggests the possibility of "parenthood by consent," including not only full recognition of adoptive parents but also gamete donation and surrogate motherhood—though he does not evaluate the desirability of such developments (*Alternatives in Jewish Bioethics* [Albany: State University of New York Press, 1997], 77–82).

66. These authorities may claim, however, that procreation removed from sex becomes more vulnerable to competing concerns; for example, it would not justify masturbation to obtain the sperm.

67. Talmud *Niddah* 31a, *Kiddushin* 30b. Other examples of humans acting as partners with God are presented in *Shabbat* 10a, 119b.

68. Bleich represents an exception; he suggests fertilizing only one ovum at a time.

69. Catholic and Jewish writers alike express concern that the use of donor gametes affects the child negatively by blurring genealogy and complicating the child's relations with his or her parents. Jewish writers are more likely to focus on the possible though unlikely risk of violating a prohibition against consanguineous marriages.

70. Or in other cases when the husband's sperm is used, as when the wife gestates and gives birth to a child arising from a donated egg.

71. Vacek, "Notes on Moral Theology," 117. Vacek and some other Catholic theologians do accord suffering more decisive weight; as a general tendency, however, such a view is more common among Jewish writers.

72. Suffering is less prominent in discussions of homologous IVF because this procedure is generally accepted even aside from consideration of suffering—although suffering is central in Nebenzal's response to Waldenberg (see note 36).

73. Dorff also notes demographic concerns, in light of the relatively small size of the Jewish community. I address this factor more fully in the Conclusion.

74. See Aaron L. Mackler, "Is There a Unique Jewish Bioethics of Human Reproduction," *Annual of the Society of Christian Ethics* 21 (2001): 319–23.

Chapter 7

Access to Health Care and Rationing

PROVISION OF HEALTH CARE REPRESENTS A CHALLENGE OF great and growing importance for contemporary societies. Whereas health care in centuries past was inexpensive but largely ineffective, in our time medicine can do remarkable things to save and enhance lives—but at considerable cost. How should that cost be apportioned, and how should societies decide what to guarantee to individual citizens? Although historically few religious thinkers addressed questions of access to health care and rationing, these newly important concerns touch on values and responsibilities that are central to Judaism and Roman Catholicism.[1]

In this chapter I examine Jewish and Roman Catholic approaches to issues of access to health care and rationing. I present and compare substantive positions, with attention to methodological approaches, as well as ways in which treatment of these issues reflects and sheds light on broader characteristics of the faith traditions. As with other issues examined in this book, to an impressive extent moral thinkers in both traditions frame the issues in similar ways and identify similar sets of specific concerns. Writers in each tradition support the guarantee of universal access to at least a basic level of health care for all members of society. This guarantee is grounded in the shared values noted in the introduction—such as the intrinsic dignity of human persons, created in the image of God; the responsibility of a just society to offer needed support to its members; and a divine mandate to provide healing to people in need. Thinkers in the two traditions express generally similar understandings of God, humanity, and the world, often citing the same scriptural texts. Catholic writers are more likely to frame their arguments in terms of the common good. Partly for this reason, Catholic writers tend to be somewhat more accepting of rationing that denies beneficial health care to some persons.

Methodologically, writers in the two traditions present similar reasoning. As with the issues examined in preceding chapters, there is some tendency for natural law and teleological arguments to be more prominent among Catholic thinkers and appeals to tradition more prominent among Jewish writers.[2] This contrast reflects general characteristics of the religions. Jewish ethics has long focused on tradition and halakhah, though reason and experience always have been part of the process as well; Catholic ethics has focused on natural law and reason, though tradition has been recognized as an important source of authority. Partly because of methodological differences, Catholic writers tend to regard application of Catholic ethics to societies such as the United States as relatively unproblematic. Teachings of natural law traditionally are understood to apply to all humans and to be accessible to all on the basis of reason. Jewish writers tend to regard application to general society of teachings based on Jewish law and traditional narratives as a more complex enterprise. In this chapter I consider briefly some possible explanations for the convergence of the traditions, as well as factors that may contribute to the differences. I also address briefly the significance of the convergence and divergence between these traditions for public policy in societies such as the United States.

Shared Values

Jewish and Catholic writers addressing issues of access to health care and rationing appeal to many of the same values (see Introduction). A foundational text in each tradition is the teaching in the book of Genesis that God created humans in God's image. This concept powerfully expresses the intrinsic value and dignity of each human being. The same verse provides a source for the commitment of each tradition to the value of human life and to the imperative to save and preserve life. Each tradition calls on its followers to love their neighbors as themselves and to pursue the path of *imitatio Dei*, following the model of God's works of mercy as described in the Hebrew Bible or the loving works of Christ. Although Jews and Catholics acknowledge God's ultimate sovereignty, they are called to exercise stewardship in acting to help other persons and to improve the world. These values support provision of health care to people in need. For both traditions, humans are essentially social. Individuals appropriately pursue their well-being as members of communities, and a flourishing community supports the well-being of its members. The good of the community as a whole represents an important value for each tradition—especially in Roman Catholicism, where it is understood in terms of the common good. Justice represents both God's will and an essential virtue for any society. It entails meeting basic material needs for all members of society, including people who are poor and vulnerable, and the opportunity for all to participate in the activities of the community.

Communal Responsibility and Access to Health Care

Writers in each tradition build on these values to argue for a societal obligation to assure at least a basic level of health care. Pope John XXIII's 1963 encyclical, *Pacem in Terris*, proclaims, "We see that every man has the right to life, to bodily integrity, and to the means which are suitable for the proper development of life," including medical care. "Therefore a human being also has the right to security in cases of sickness."[3] This right to health care is developed in the U.S. bishops' "Pastoral Letter on Health and Health Care" of 1981, which insists as well on the individual's obligation to promote his or her own health. "Because all human beings are created according to God's image, they possess a basic human dignity which calls for the utmost reverence. On the individual level this means a special responsibility to care for one's own health and that of others. On the societal level this calls for responsibility by society to provide adequate health care which is a basic human right."[4] The first of six principles that the bishops set forth for public policy affirms the following:

> Every person has a basic right to adequate health care. This right flows from the sanctity of human life and the dignity that belongs to all human persons, who are made in the image of God. It implies that access to that health care which is necessary and suitable for the proper development and maintenance of life must be provided for all people, regardless of economic, social, or legal status. Special attention should be given to meeting the basic health needs of the poor.[5]

Another principle specifies that "the benefits provided in a national health-care policy should be sufficient to maintain and promote good health as well as to treat disease and disability." Additional principles affirm the values of pluralism, consumer choice, planning, and cost control. The bishops call for a national health insurance program and advocate an "essential role" for government and for private institutions (and the Catholic Church and its members). This inclusive approach reflects the principle of subsidiarity, which holds that individuals and smaller groups should do as much as they are able and that the larger society is responsible to step in to provide support when such support is required.[6]

More specific guidance for public policy is offered in the bishops' 1993 "Resolution on Health Care Reform." The bishops appeal to the affirmations of the foregoing documents, as well as "the biblical call to heal the sick and to serve 'the least of these,' the priorities of social justice and the principle of the common good." These principles are joined with notions of the values of solidarity and stewardship. The bishops endorse "comprehensive reform that will ensure a decent level of health care for all without regard to their ability to pay," again with government playing an "essential role" in conjunction with private providers; they propose eight criteria for reform. Commitments to universal access, comprehensive benefits, pluralism, and cost containment embody principles articulated in the earlier Pastoral Letter. These commitments are joined by explicit attention to "respect for life" ("from conception to natural death"), priority concern for poor people, assurance of quality in care, and "equitable financing." (The earlier document's principles of planning and consumer choice have receded to the background.) In addition to making policy recommendations, the bishops note the importance of appropriate attitudes, recognizing that "we are all called to protect human life, promote human dignity and pursue the common good."[7]

On the general issue of access to health care, the magisterial statements represent points of broad consensus among Roman Catholic thinkers. Lisa Sowle Cahill and Andrew Lustig suggest that the bishops may not be sufficiently realistic about the difficulty of achieving their goals and the likely need for tradeoffs among their principles.[8] Richard McCormick questions the advisability of a national health insurance plan that is likely to maintain the U.S. orientation toward curative care and high technology.[9] All agree, however, on the responsibility of society to assure health care for all of its members, grounded in the values of human dignity, justice, and the common good.

Judaism does not have a centralized authority analogous to the Roman Catholic magisterium or the National Conference of Bishops. Nor does it have the same tradition of documents arguing from general premises to normative guidelines. As I have noted in preceding chapters, the tradition's dominant mode of addressing particular issues is the development of halakhic responsa by individual rabbinic authorities, addressing particular cases and issues brought to their attention. The model is similar to that of U.S. case law or the (classical and contemporary) casuistry advocated by Albert Jonsen and others.[10] General values are present but may remain implicit or appear only in passing, embedded in precedent cases and narratives of the tradition. In recent years, this literature has been supplemented by scholarly analyses developed by individual thinkers and by formal resolutions adopted by various groups.

With all of these caveats, Jewish authorities overwhelmingly agree with the consensus of their Catholic counterparts that society has a responsibility to assure health care for all of its members. This position is supported by the tradition's powerful mandate for the provision of healing.[11] The commitment flows as well from traditional values and practices of *tzedakah*—a word meaning justice and referring to support for poor people—assuring the basic needs of individuals in society.[12]

Within Orthodox (right-wing) Judaism, Rabbi Eliezer Yehudah Waldenberg rules that when an individual cannot afford to pay for needed medical care, society acquires the obligation to assure that person's treatment.[13] Waldenberg's ruling and this general principle are affirmed by thinkers such as Rabbi J. David Bleich and Fred Rosner, who proclaims that "universal access to health care is a moral imperative based in part on traditional Judeo-Christian ethics."[14] In 1991 the Reform (left-wing) Central Conference of American Rabbis adopted a resolution that "we seek a national health plan which grants universal access to health care benefits." "A broadly shared concern for justice" provides the basis for this proposal. A list of twelve criteria for the desired national health plan overlaps significantly with lists of the National Conference of Catholic Bishops, presented before and after this resolution. These criteria include "serv[ing] everyone living in the United States"; "comprehensive benefits, including: preventive services and health promotion, primary and acute care, mental health care, and extended care"; broad-based financial support; quality; cost containment; "a national budget for health education and wellness promotion"; and "federal leadership in health promotion by assessing the health impacts of standard of living issues, housing, nutrition, physical fitness, environmental safety, and sanitation."[15]

A responsum approved by the Committee on Jewish Law and Standards of the Conservative (centrist) movement likewise appeals to values such as respect for persons, justice, healing, and the saving of life:

> Jewish law requires that people be provided with needed health care, at least a "decent minimum" that preserves life and meets other basic needs, including some amount of preventive care. The responsibility to assure this provision is shared among individuals and families, physicians and other health care providers, and the community. Individuals and family members have the responsibility to care for their own health, and the primary responsibility to pay (directly or through insurance) for health care needed by themselves or by family members. . . . The community bears ultimate responsibility to assure provision of needed health care for individuals who cannot afford it, as a matter of justice as well as a specific halakhic obligation.[16]

Authors in both traditions agree that individuals are not entitled to unlimited health care, and societies cannot be expected to provide any medical intervention that any individual might desire. Most commonly, the standard for the health care that must be provided is that of need. For example, in the Catholic tradition, Joseph Boyle argues as follows:

> Different criteria are no doubt appropriate for distributing different goods, but in the case of health care the appropriate criterion seems to be need. Need is the basis for the informal obligation everyone has to help his or her sick neighbor. . . . So, a person has a right to those health care services he or she reasonably needs and which can be provided within a system which can provide for the similar needs of others.[17]

According to the bishops' Pastoral Letter, "access to that health care which is necessary and suitable for the proper development and maintenance of life must be provided for all people." The bishops' "Resolution on Health Care Reform" argues that "genuine health care reform must especially focus on the basic health needs of the poor"; the resolution insists on "comprehensive benefits sufficient to maintain and promote good health, to provide preventive care, to treat disease, injury and disability appropriately."[18] Jewish thinkers argue likewise:

> The standard for the amount of care to be assured is that of need. Patients are not entitled to, and society is not obligated to provide, all care that is desired, all care that might offer some benefit, or all care that anyone else in the society receives. The community is obligated, however, to assure access to all care that is needed by a patient to lead a reasonably full life. While identifying "needed" treatments will change with developing medical practice and vary among individual cases, in general it would be treatment that would be effective in sustaining life, curing disease, restoring health, or improving function.[19]

For Catholic and Jewish writers alike, society has an important responsibility to assure the provision of needed health care to all.

Limits and Rationing: The Extent of Communal Responsibility to Assure Access to Care

Are there limits on society's obligation to assure all care that patients need? Thinkers in each tradition acknowledge that there could be. Societies have other obligations that may compete for resources, including provision of adequate food and shelter, education, and maintaining public order.[20] Society also has a responsibility to plan to meet future needs, which could justify allocating some resources to preventive care and research, even at the expense of some acute treatment for patients currently in need.[21]

Within this general consensus, some divergent tendencies between Catholic and Jewish thinkers are evident. These differences are matters of degree and tend to be relatively minor in comparison to the overall agreement between the traditions. Moreover, there is a range of views within each tradition. Nevertheless, there is some tendency for Catholic thinkers to be less willing than their Jewish counterparts to diminish aid for individuals who are responsible for their own illness; to be more insistent on maintaining equality through a "single tier" system that provides the same care to all members of society; and to accept rationing that denies beneficial, and even needed, care.

Thinkers in both traditions express compassion for persons who are responsible in part for their illness, as well as appreciation for their intrinsic dignity and the value of their lives. Jewish authors are somewhat more ready, however, to declare that in cases of absolute scarcity in which needed care must be denied to some persons, it is fair to accord higher priority to those who did not contribute to their own illness. Conservative rabbi Elliot Dorff argues,

> However we identify vital communal services in our own day, since no community's resources are limitless, each one must ensure that those who receive public assistance for health care deserve it. Thus if a person repeatedly endangers his or her health through practices—such as smoking, drug or alcohol abuse, or overeating—known to constitute major risks, the community may decide to impose a limit on the public resources that such a person can call upon to finance the curative procedures she or he needs as a consequence of these unhealthy habits.[22]

The community should give a second chance to individuals who make unwise choices and provide some degree of care to all in need, but a lesser degree of assistance may be appropriate. Such limits are supported by the value of justice and by texts limiting the obligations of the community to redeem an individual who has sold himself into captivity or a criminal who is endangering the safety of a community in which he seeks shelter.[23] In contrast, the Catholic Health Association (CHA), in a document arguing for appropriate rationing of health care, insists that "when people are in need of healthcare services, the way they contracted their disease and the extent to which they may be personally responsible must play *no part* in decisions to withhold healthcare services."[24]

Catholic writers tend to emphasize the importance of everybody receiving equal care, in a one-tier system. The bishops' Resolution argues that "true universal access" is not compatible with "a two-tiered system since separate health care coverage for the poor usually results in poor health care."[25] Cardinal Joseph Bernadin adds a concern that such an approach "marginalizes large portions of our society" and detracts from the value of solidarity.[26] The Catholic Health Association insists that "rationing should apply to all."

> Healthcare rationing must promote and not undermine this sense of social solidarity that makes the realization of human dignity possible. Only when rationing applies to all can it be the occasion for sharing a common hardship rather than an occasion for deepening the gaps between wealthy and poor, old and young, healthy and sick, and among racial groups. Equity in rationing would suffer if a significant minority of the public obtained their care outside the healthcare system while acquiescing to limitations on services for those who were economically less secure.[27]

Although Jewish writers also are committed to the value of equality, they tend to be less concerned with maintaining a single-tier system. They would agree on the need for a floor to assure a basic minimum of care for all, but they would not see a need for a ceiling to keep everyone on the same level. In part this acceptance of different levels is practical and reflects the right of individuals to use their resources for their own benefit (after having discharged their communal obligations).[28] In addition, this freedom to spend more on health care reflects the value accorded to healing. Devoting large amounts of one's resources to strengthening the body and preserving the life that God has given in trust is commendable.

The divergence between the traditions on this issue is far from absolute. All agree on values of healing and equality. Furthermore, although official Catholic documents consistently insist on a single tier, individual moral theologians may be more flexible. In analyzing the bishops' resolution, Catholic scholar Andrew Lustig notes,

> The potential for tensions between a commitment to a single-tiered system and a respect for pluralism of individuals and institutions is enormous. Moreover, in light of the theological convictions central to the broader Catholic discussion of health care, considerations of individual liberty and dignity, as well as the common good, might reasonably lead to a different practical conclusion; viz., that two tiers

of health care delivery are morally appropriate and practically preferable, so long as universal access to comprehensive basic care is assured.[29]

Finally, there is some divergence with regard to the willingness of thinkers in each tradition to accept rationing that denies patients beneficial health care (or fails to provide such care). Jewish thinkers tend to be less willing to accept rationing, though again the difference is one of degree. Jewish thinkers agree that resources may be limited, calling for difficult decisions on allocation.[30] Catholic writers typically argue that "the need for healthcare rationing must be demonstrable. Because it can threaten the health or even lives of individuals, healthcare rationing requires strong ethical justification."[31] Nonetheless, Jewish writers tend to be more reluctant, and Catholic writers more ready, to endorse rationing for contemporary U.S. society.

The Catholic Health Association (CHA), for example, accepts rationing—defined as "the withholding of potentially beneficial services because policies and practices establish limits on the resources available for healthcare." It argues that de facto rationing, denying services to poor people, occurs currently and notes that proposals for explicit rationing have been made, in Oregon and elsewhere. "These systemic attempts to deny people access to potentially beneficial services suggest a need for a set of ethical criteria by which current and proposed forms of rationing can be evaluated." The CHA proposes eight criteria: "the need for healthcare rationing must be demonstrable"; "healthcare rationing must be oriented to the common good"; "a basic level of healthcare must be available to all"; "rationing should apply to all"; "rationing must result from an open, participatory process"; "the healthcare of disadvantaged persons has an ethical priority"; "rationing must be free of wrongful discrimination"; and "the social and economic effects of healthcare rationing must be monitored." A system of rationing may be justified even if it does not meet all of these criteria, as long as it represents an improvement over current practices.[32]

Similar views are widely shared among Catholic thinkers. Cardinal Bernadin argues that rationing, as defined by the CHA, is "an issue of balance between the individual and the community, both of which have acknowledged needs. Under this definition, we do not prejudge the issue of whether a specific proposal or method of rationing is good or evil; we leave open the possibility that withholding care may be justified by limits on resources."[33] Philip Keane proposes a list of criteria that would justify rationing—similar to the list offered by the CHA—and argues that rationing must be accepted.[34]

Although Jewish thinkers agree in general with claims about human finitude and limits of resources, they tend to be more reluctant to endorse rationing as a current policy choice.[35] For example, the Conservative movement responsum argues that "rationing that denies needed care is a last resort, and at best premature, given the lack of serious efforts to provide needed care or to limit that which is unneeded."[36] Laurie Zoloth expresses appreciation for the Oregon Health Care Decision Making Project and endorses the value of communal solidarity. Nonetheless, she rejects rationing.

> As long as rationing focuses on the limitation of care and not the limitation of profits, it will continue to burden the most vulnerable disproportionately, shifting the cost of the solution onto those individuals least able to bear it. Justly to address the problem of limits will mean subjecting to scrutiny each aspect of the medical system, not simply the appropriate limits of a basic decent minimum health care package.[37]

Differences between Jewish and Catholic writers could reflect, in part, different uses of the term *rationing*. Philosopher Daniel Wikler helpfully distinguishes among "three grades of rationing": "Rationing as Trimming is cutting back on services that few people want and no one needs." Cutting, or "hard rationing," means "refusing genuinely needed and wanted care on the grounds that the cost is 'too high.'" Tailoring is intermediate—denying treatments of questionable effectiveness that people may want but not truly need or treatment that is effective in prolonging marginally endurable existence but that most patients would choose not to receive.[38] To the extent that Catholic writers are endorsing rationing as trimming or tailoring and Jewish writers are rejecting rationing as cutting, they would not be disagreeing substantively. Nevertheless, it would be significant that Catholic writers choose to focus on an endorsement of good rationing and Jewish writers on opposing bad rationing. There is at least a difference in rhetoric and emphasis between a position that proclaims that "of course some limits are unavoidable, but rationing must be a last resort," and one that proclaims, "of course rationing should be a last resort, but limits are unavoidable."

Acknowledging these caveats, it remains true that to a significant extent, Catholic writers are relatively willing to accept rationing for current U.S. policy, and Jewish writers are reluctant to do so. Several possible reasons could be suggested. To at least some degree, the Jewish tradition tends to understand the provision of needed health care, and support for the poor generally, as a perfect obligation, which must be met fully in every case; on the other hand, the Catholic tradition tends to view such aid as an imperfect obligation—which must be pursued, but without the same demand that every need be met. As Wikler frames the issue, advocates of hard rationing claim that "we must swallow the bitter pill of Cutting and revise our conventional thinking about the moral imperative to use all the medical means we have developed to save the sick."[39] This claim is even more difficult to make in the Jewish tradition than in the Catholic tradition. Although the terms should be used with caution, Jewish ethics (on this topic, at least) tends to be deontological in its formulation, so provision of needed health care is a societal duty in each case. Catholic ethics tends to be teleological (especially with regard to positive duties), so society should work generally to pursue the good of the provision of needed care, but without quite the same urgency in every case.

For each tradition, provision of needed care combines justice and mercy; for Catholicism, however, mercy is more dominant. The word *charity* is derived from a word meaning "love." Healing is an example of the corporal works of mercy. "The works of mercy call Christians to engage themselves in direct efforts to alleviate the misery of the afflicted."[40] In Judaism, the word *tzedakah* is related to a word meaning "justice," *tzedek*. Although ideally *tzedakah* would be given with compassion, the basic requirement to give a fixed percentage of income is legally enforceable. In Jewish tradition, provision of basic needs is guaranteed to poor people by the community, as a matter of justice and right.[41]

Similarly, each tradition accords value both to individuals and to the community as a whole. Relative to Judaism, Catholicism tends to shift the balance a little more to the side of the common good.[42] The common good is the "good for society as a whole which respects but is ultimately more important than the good of any individual."[43] For the common good to be achieved, support must be given to individuals in general, and individuals in general must be able to participate as active members of society. Accordingly, when a balance must be reached between liberty and the good of some individuals, on one hand, and equality and solidarity on the other, the balance will tilt somewhat toward equality and solidarity. Cutting care that is needed by some individuals, to enrich the community in a way that on the whole helps most individuals, could be acceptable.

Furthermore, although each tradition values physical life, it tends to play a more decisive role in Judaism. A typical Jewish understanding is that this world and life eternal represent two goods that are each basic and incommensurable, neither serving only instrumentally for the other. Preservation of life, *pikuaḥ nefesh*, is decisive in virtually every case. For many Catholic theologians, preservation of life in this world is less of an absolute imperative. The central narrative of Jesus's death and resurrection has relativized the life of this world, which is subordinated to spiritual development and life eternal.[44] After defining the common good as "embracing the sum total of those conditions of social living whereby men are enabled to achieve their own integral perfection more fully and more easily," the encyclical *Pacem in Terris* continues, "Men, however, composed as they are of bodies and immortal souls, can never in this mortal life succeed in satisfying all their needs or in attaining perfect happiness. Therefore the common good is to be procured by such ways and means which not only are not detrimental to man's eternal salvation but which positively contribute to it."[45] Although the common good would not justify unjustly killing an individual, pursuit of the common good might take priority over efforts to save individual lives. As an illustration of the difference in temperaments, Catholic thinker Keane suggests that because "we have been unable to develop a prejudice-free process for allocating scarce organs . . . it might be morally better not to transplant scarce organs until we can find a truly moral process for allocating them."[46] Although Jewish writers would support the importance of fighting prejudice and morally improving the allocation system, it would be hard to find one who would advocate allowing preventable deaths until a more perfect system is achieved.

Given these general orientations, it makes sense that Judaism tends to accord some greater priority to aiding patients who are not responsible for their illness because they are owed such support as a matter of justice. Those who are responsible for their own illness should be given treatment because of mercy and respect for intrinsic human dignity, but they would have a lesser claim in a forced-choice situation. Catholics would be more likely to insist on a single-tier system, which would strengthen the community through values of equality and solidarity, whereas Judaism would be more supportive of individuals vigorously pursuing their healing and preservation of life. Catholics would be more likely to accept denial of needed care to some individuals, in the context of strengthening the overall community, whereas Jews would be more reluctant to deny needed care to any individual in the name of the common good. Nevertheless, one should keep in mind that these differences represent relatively minor variations in the context of the common ground that Jewish and Catholic writers share to an impressive extent.

Public Policy

Jewish and Catholic writers alike present their statements as important for public policy in societies such as the United States. The bishops' 1981 Pastoral Letter is addressed to Catholics. It aims "to call all Catholics to a fuller acceptance of their responsibility for their own health and for their share in the healing apostolate of the church" and to "provide a sound framework for an ongoing discussion of health and healing in the American Catholic community." The Catholic understandings developed thereby will indirectly have implications for national policy. "We will offer some basic principles for public policy as a means of encouraging full and responsible participation by Catholics in the shaping of national health policies." Again, the bishops assert that "Christian people have a responsibility to actively participate in the shaping and executing of public policy that relates to health care. On this issue, as on all issues of basic human rights, the church has an important role to play in bringing gospel values to the social and political order."[47]

The 1993 "Resolution on Health Care Reform" seeks more direct application to U.S. policy. It is addressed "to the Catholic community *and the leaders of our nation.*" Accordingly, the document restricts itself to natural law reasoning, making ethical appeals grounded in human experience and the nature of the human person. In the pastoral letter the model of Jesus's healing is prominent. In contrast, the resolution does not explicitly include the words "Jesus" or "gospel" (although there is one general reference to "the biblical call to heal the sick and to serve 'the least of these'").[48] Why the difference in tone? In part it simply may reflect the narrower scope of the Resolution. The pastoral letter addresses health care generally, with extensive discussion of "the healing apostolate of the church." The resolution focuses on the aspect of health care that is involved in national policy. The difference also may reflect a growing confidence that the Catholic natural law tradition can speak directly to all Americans and to all human persons. Between the 1981 letter and 1993 resolution, the bishops had issued their 1983 pastoral letter, "The Challenge of Peace," and their 1986 letter, "Economic Justice for All"—both of which attracted discussion in general U.S. society.[49]

Jewish writers are less likely to make claims about universal human morality. Orthodox writers in particular are hesitant to extrapolate, from the requirements that Jewish law and ethics mandate for a traditional Jewish community, to a secular nation state. Even within Orthodoxy there are exceptions, as in Rosner's statement that "universal access to health care is a moral imperative based in part on traditional Judeo-Christian ethics."[50] Other Jewish writers are more ready to address the implications of Jewish ethics for general society, especially when these ethical principles are based on justice, as noted in the Reform rabbis' resolution. The Conservative responsum articulates a stance similar to that in the bishops' 1981 pastoral letter.

> Specific claims of halakhah are not binding on secular nations, of course. Jewish understandings of justice should not (and could not) be imposed monolithically, but should contribute to a national dialogue in which diverse philosophical, religious, and other views would be represented. In the Jewish understanding developed in this paper, securing access to all health care that is needed represents a matter of foundational justice. And whatever the differences between

traditional Jewish societies and contemporary countries such as the United States and Canada, all societies are appropriately responsible for the achievement of foundational justice. Jews who are citizens of democratic societies have at least some degree of responsibility to support general institutions that will assure the provision of needed care, through lobbying, social action, and other means.[51]

Roman Catholic and Jewish perspectives offer important contributions to ethical and policy deliberations in countries such as the United States. As Lisa Sowle Cahill has observed, public policy discourse on bioethical issues "is actually a meeting ground of the diverse moral traditions that make up our society." Religious and secular traditions alike contribute to this discourse, making distinctive contributions both when they articulate shared commitments and when they offer differing perspectives.[52] The shared Roman Catholic and Jewish understanding of the responsibility to assure access to at least a basic level of health care to all members of society stakes out important common ground. This agreement could be part of an overlapping consensus shared across divergent worldviews. Societal responsibility to assure access to care could represent a "locus of certitude" that diverse individuals and groups could support, even if they provide differing rationales for this shared commitment.[53] As Cahill notes, writings developed within a given religious tradition may support ethical positions that could be justified on other secular or religious grounds. "Consensus in and about the public order is contingent not on genuine universality, but on intelligibility and persuasiveness within a community of communities."[54]

Such a consensus could be politically important in the development of governmental policy, which supports the feasibility of such a position. It certainly would represent a powerful articulation of the shared values and commitments of society. In addition, the consensus may have a deeper significance in strengthening the warranted status of the belief that access to health care ought to be assured.[55]

Cahill notes that theological traditions contribute to public discourse not only when they articulate shared views but also when they offer a countercultural critical perspective, challenging widely held assumptions. Within their general common-ground affirmation of a societal obligation to assure the provision of health care to all its members, the Jewish and Roman Catholic traditions have complementary perspectives and strengths. With regard to the desire for a single tier of health care that all members of society share, Jewish writers may be more realistic, acknowledging competing values of liberty and beneficence, as well as concerns for practical feasibility. The Catholic perspective provides a critical prophetic voice, emphasizing the values of equality and solidarity and warning us not to be too comfortable with the gaps in our society. With regard to rationing, Catholic writers may be more realistic, recognizing that limits in the provision of health care are unavoidable. Here the Jewish perspective provides a critical prophetic voice, emphasizing the value of each individual person. We should not be too comfortable in denying needed care to any individual.

Notes

1. This paragraph is adapted from Elliot N. Dorff and Aaron L. Mackler, "Responsibilities for the Provision of Health Care," in *Life and Death Responsibilities in Jewish Biomedical Ethics*, ed. Aaron L. Mackler (New York: Finkelstein Institute and Jewish Theological Seminary Press, 2000), 479.

2. Catholic approaches tend to be teleological in the sense of understanding the ends of the human person and human society to be foundational in ethical deliberation, not necessarily in the sense of consequentialism often associated with this term. See Benedict M. Ashley and Kevin D. O'Rourke, *Health Care Ethics: A Theological Analysis*, 4th ed. (Washington, D.C.: Georgetown University Press, 1997), 156–66, and the discussion in chapter 1.

3. *Peace on Earth [Pacem in Terris]* (Washington, D.C.: National Catholic Welfare Conference, 1963), n. 11, p. 5. The language of "rights" is found frequently in Roman Catholic discourse on this topic; it is rare among Jewish writers, who prefer the language of responsibility and obligation. This difference does not seem to affect the substantive positions of writers in the two traditions. In fact, as I note, Jewish thinkers are more likely to understand there to be a perfect obligation to provide needed health care—a position that is more likely to correlate with a patient's right to receive care.

4. National Conference of Catholic Bishops, "Pastoral Letter on Health and Health Care," *Origins* 11 (1981): 397–98.

5. Ibid., 402.

6. Ibid.; James P. Hanigan, *As I Have Loved You: The Challenge of Christian Ethics* (Mahwah, N.J.: Paulist, 1986), 82–83.

7. National Conference of Catholic Bishops, "Resolution on Health Care Reform," *Origins* 23 (1993): 98–102. The same set of criteria, in a different order, appeared in the bishops' "Criteria for Evaluating Health Care Reform," *Origins* 22 (1992): 23–24.

8. Lisa Sowle Cahill, "Good News and Bad," *Health Progress* 80, no. 4 (1999): 18–23; B. Andrew Lustig, "The Common Good in a Secular Society: The Relevance of a Roman Catholic Notion to the Healthcare Allocation Debate," *Journal of Medicine and Philosophy* 18 (1983): 569–87; idem, "Reform and Rationing: Reflections on Health Care in Light of Catholic Social Teaching," in *Secular Bioethics in Theological Perspectives*, ed. Earl E. Shelp (Dordrecht, Netherlands: Kluwer, 1996), 31–50.

9. Richard A. McCormick, "A Catholic Perspective on Access to Care," *Cambridge Quarterly of Healthcare Ethics* 7 (1998): 254–59. See also Philip S. Keane, *Health Care Reform: A Catholic View* (New York: Paulist, 1993); Joseph M. Boyle, "The Right to Health Care and Its Limits," in *Scarce Medical Resources and Justice*, ed. Pope John XXIII Medical-Moral Research and Education Center (Braintree, Mass.: Pope John XXIII Medical-Moral Research and Education Center, 1987), 13–25; Charles J. Dougherty, *Back to Reform: Values, Markets and the Health Care System* (New York: Oxford University Press, 1996). Catholic physician Edmund D. Pellegrino advocates a value of "charitable justice," which "would mean equity in distribution of essential services regardless of ability to pay. It entails universal accessibility to health care without discrimination. On this view, health care becomes an obligation of the whole Christian community because charitable justice recognizes a moral claim on all of us by the sick, disabled, poor, and rejected members of our society" (Edmund Pellegrino, "Healing and Being Healed: A Christian Perspective," in *Jewish and Catholic Bioethics: An Ecumenical Dialogue*, ed. Edmund D. Pellegrino and Alan I. Faden [Washington, D.C.: Georgetown University Press, 1999], 123).

10. Albert R. Jonsen and Stephen Toulmin, *The Abuse of Casuistry: A History of Moral Reasoning* (Berkeley: University of California Press, 1988). See also the discussion in chapter 2.

11. David M. Feldman, *Health and Medicine in the Jewish Tradition* (New York: Crossroad, 1986), 15–27; Fred Rosner, *Modern Medicine and Jewish Ethics*, 2d ed. (Hoboken, N.J.: Ktav, 1991), 5–19. The mandate to heal traditionally is grounded in biblical commandments to heal the injured (Exodus 21:19); to restore that which has been lost—construed to include lost health and function (Deuteronomy 22:2); not to stand idly by the blood of

one's neighbor (Leviticus 19:16); and to love one's neighbor as oneself (Leviticus 19:18).

12. Aaron L. Mackler, "Judaism, Justice, and Access to Health Care," *Kennedy Institute of Ethics Journal* 1 (1991): 143–61.

13. Eliezer Yehudah Waldenberg, *Ramat Raḥel*, no. 24, in *Tzitz Eliezer*, 2d ed. (Jerusalem: n.p., 1985), v. 5, pp. 31–32.

14. J. David Bleich, *Judaism and Healing* (New York: Ktav, 1981), 13–16; Fred Rosner, "Managed Care: A Contradiction or Fulfillment of Jewish Law? ftp://ftp.ijme.org/pub/Transcripts/Rosner/rmanagedcare.txt (accessed April 16, 1998; no longer available). According to Orthodox rabbi Moshe Tendler, "On the Interface of Religion and Medical Science: The Judeo-Biblical Perspective," in Pellegrino and Faden, *Jewish and Catholic Bioethics*, 107 (quoting Leviticus 19:16), "The duty to provide for medical care for all is imposed on nonphysicians as well [as physicians] by the commandment: 'You shall not stand idly by' which is interpreted as requiring the expenditure of funds to provide medical care for the indigent. This is the ethical basis for universal health insurance."

15. Central Conference of American Rabbis (CCAR), "National Health Care," resolution adopted by the CCAR, June 1991; www.ccarnet.org/cgi-bin/resodisp.pl?file=care&year=1991.

16. Dorff and Mackler, "Responsibilities for the Provision of Health Care," 499–500. The endorsement of the Rabbinical Assembly's Committee on Jewish Law and Standards reflects authorization beyond the individual views of the authors of the paper.

17. Boyle, "The Right to Health Care," 22.

18. National Conference of Catholic Bishops, "Pastoral Letter," 402; "Resolution on Health Care Reform," 100.

19. Dorff and Mackler, "Responsibilities for the Provision of Health Care," 493.

20. Boyle, "The Right to Health Care," 22; Joseph Bernadin, "The Consistent Ethic of Life and Health Care Reform," *Origins* 24 (1994): 60–64; Elliot N. Dorff, *Matters of Life and Death: A Jewish Approach to Modern Medical Ethics* (Philadelphia: Jewish Publication Society, 1998), 281–88; Laurie Zoloth, *Health Care and the Ethics of Encounter: A Jewish Discussion of Social Justice* (Chapel Hill: University of North Carolina Press, 1999), 189–92.

21. Martin P. Golding, "Preventive vs. Curative Medicine: Perspectives of the Jewish Legal Tradition," *Journal of Medicine and Philosophy* 8 (1983): 269–86; Noam J. Zohar, *Alternatives in Jewish Bioethics* (Albany: State University of New York Press, 1997), 143–52.

22. Dorff, *Matters of Life and Death*, 303.

23. Ibid., 303–4.

24. Catholic Health Association of the United States, *With Justice for All? The Ethics of Healthcare Rationing* (St. Louis: Catholic Health Association of the United States, 1991), 25; emphasis added.

25. National Conference of Catholic Bishops, "Resolution on Health Care Reform," 100–101.

26. Bernadin, "Consistent Ethic of Life," 62.

27. Catholic Health Association, *With Justice for All?* 22–23.

28. A legal precedent involves the redemption of captives—those captured by slave traders or unjustly held prisoner. The community generally does not ransom individuals for more than their fair market value—in part to discourage the capture of more hostages—but an individual may choose to pay more than that to free himself or family members. See Dorff, *Matters of Life and Death*, 305.

29. Lustig, "Reform and Rationing," 41. See also David F. Kelly, *Critical Care Ethics: Treatment Decisions in American Hospitals* (Kansas City, Mo.: Sheed and Ward, 1991), 153. Catholic philosopher Charles Dougherty, *Back to Reform*, 120–21, likewise argues that a two-tier system could be acceptable, in light of competing values and practical considerations.

30. Avraham Steinberg observes that no society is able to provide all needed health care for all of its citizens (*Encyclopedia of Jewish Medical Ethics,* vol. 4 [Jerusalem: Schlesinger Institute, 1988], s.v. "Limited Resources," 245, 249). Daniel Eisenberg writes that "rationing of medical care is not intrinsically problematic. There are established principles in Jewish law regarding triage" ("Is Managed Care Unethical?" *Maimonides* 3, no. 2 [1997]: 3).

31. Catholic Health Association, *With Justice for All?* 19.

32. Ibid., ix–xi, 19–26.

33. Joseph Bernadin, "Managing Managed Care," *Origins* 26 (1996): 24.

34. Keane, *Health Care Reform*, 144–48, 188–91.

35. Some people might consider according a lower priority to individuals who contributed to their own illness, as discussed above, to be a form of rationing—perhaps rationing by merit or by dessert. Jewish authors who accept such prioritizing tend to distinguish this concept from rationing. Secular philosopher Norman Daniels observes that "when we ration, we deny benefits to some individuals who can plausibly claim that they are owed them in principle. They can cite an accepted principle of distributive justice that governs their situation and should protect them" ("Rationing Fairly: Programmatic Considerations," *Bioethics* 7 [1993]: 224). For authors who would allow consideration of responsibility for illness in prioritizing access to

care, patients who contribute to their own illness lessen their claim to resources. Although resources should be provided when possible as a matter of beneficence, they are not owed strictly as a matter of justice, so denial of resources on this basis would be distinct from general forms of rationing.

36. Dorff and Mackler, "Responsibilities for the Provision of Health Care," 504.

37. Zoloth, *Health Care and the Ethics of Encounter*, 233. Most Catholic thinkers probably would agree with calls to limit unneeded care and to examine all aspects of the health care system. As a group, however, they are somewhat more willing than their Jewish counterparts to endorse rationing at the present time.

38. Daniel Wikler, "Ethics and Rationing: 'Whether,' 'How,' or 'How Much?'" *Journal of the American Geriatrics Society* 40 (1992): 398–403.

39. Ibid., 401.

40. Boyle, "The Right to Health Care," 15; National Conference of Catholic Bishops, "Pastoral Letter," 398.

41. See Mackler, "Judaism, Justice, and Access to Health Care," 145–47.

42. The difference in balance is relatively minor. Catholic writers accord important value to each individual human person, and Jewish writers acknowledge the importance of the community (see Steinberg, *Encyclopedia of Jewish Medical Ethics*, vol. 4, 261; and Zoloth, *Health Care and the Ethics of Encounter*).

43. Keane, *Health Care Reform*, 130.

44. See discussions in Introduction and Conclusion.

45. John XXIII, *Pacem in Terris*, nn. 58–59, p. 16.

46. Keane, *Health Care Reform*, 189.

47. National Conference of Catholic Bishops, "Pastoral Letter," 397, 401.

48. National Conference of Catholic Bishops, "Resolution on Health Care Reform," 97, 99 (emphasis added).

49. National Conference of Catholic Bishops, *The Challenge of Peace: God's Promise and Our Response* (Washington, D.C.: United States Catholic Conference, 1983); *Economic Justice for All: Pastoral Letter on Catholic Social Teaching and the U.S. Economy* (Washington, D.C.: United States Catholic Conference, 1986).

50. Rosner, "Managed Care."

51. Dorff and Mackler, "Responsibilities for the Provision of Health Care," 498.

52. Lisa Sowle Cahill, "Can Theology Have a Role in 'Public' Bioethical Discourse?" *Hastings Center Report*, 20, no. 3 (1990, supp.): 11. Developments in philosophy as well as in society have led to an increased awareness

that all moral reasoning occurs within a particular context and reflects a particular tradition. There is no available neutral space of "just plain ethics" that can be pursued in a purely objective manner, abstracting from all particular viewpoints such as Judaism or Roman Catholicism. See Cahill, "Can Theology Have a Role"; Lustig, "Common Good in a Secular Society," 569–71, 585–86; Mackler, "Introduction," in *Life and Death Responsibilities*, 5, and discussion in Conclusion.

53. Jonsen and Toulmin, *Abuse of Casuistry*, 16–19.

54. Cahill, "Can Theology Have a Role," 13.

55. See Mackler, "Judaism, Justice, and Access to Health Care," 155, and discussion in Conclusion.

Conclusion

IN THE PRECEDING CHAPTERS I HAVE SURVEYED JEWISH AND Roman Catholic approaches to methodology generally, along with views on five specific issues in bioethics: euthanasia and assisted suicide, treatment decisions near the end of life, abortion, in vitro fertilization, and access to health care and rationing. This survey has disclosed important common ground between Jewish and Roman Catholic approaches to bioethics in method and substance and has sought to clarify the extent and topography of this common ground. Theologians in the two traditions share many basic values. They generally express similar understandings of God, humanity, and the world, often citing the same scriptural texts. There also are important points of divergence, including basic methodological focus; even here, however, the differences are less clear-cut than they might at first seem. Although Jewish ethics has long focused on tradition and halakhah, reason and experience have always been part of the process as well; although Catholic ethics has focused on natural law and reason, tradition has been recognized as an important source of authority. An overlapping Scripture, read in similar ways, plays a similar role in both traditions. And in recent decades, some theologians in each faith community have explored the development of moral method, often in dialogue with views from outside the faith community.

These basic similarities account for much of the common ground on particular issues. Moral deliberation in response to new bioethical challenges often is a matter of judgment, entailing practical reason to balance competing considerations and concretize the demands of general principles such as love of neighbor.[1] Theologians within each tradition have come to differing judgments on the most appropriate balances and concretizations, yielding in each a spectrum of responses. Because these judgments are based on many of the same values and concerns, the spectra overlap to a significant degree. As James Gustafson notes in comparing Catholic and Protestant approaches to ethics, a liberal (or moderate or conservative) may have more in common with a thinker of similar inclinations in another tradition than he or she would with a thinker of different leanings in the same faith tradition.[2] For example, on the issue of in vitro fertilization, Richard McCormick has more in common with J. David Bleich than he does with *Donum Vitae*, and Bleich has more in common with McCormick than he does with more liberal Jewish thinkers. The common ground includes not only judgments about which practices are appropriate but also the articulation of similar ethical concerns, often expressed in similar terms. This overlap of ranges of views is a striking outcome of this comparison.

At the same time, it is notable that the spectra of views, though overlapping, are shifted. On end-of-life decisions, the range of Jewish positions tends to overlap with and extend somewhat to the right of Catholic views—expressing greater reluctance to forgo life-sustaining treatment; on in vitro fertilization and abortion, the Catholic range overlaps and extends somewhat to the right of Jewish views, expressing greater reluctance to allow these procedures. To take the same theologians as markers, Bleich would occupy a centrist position among Catholic views on IVF but would be off the scale to the right in restricting decisions near the end of life. McCormick's position would be right of center on the scale of Jewish views on IVF but would be at the left edge in authorizing decisions to stop life-sustaining treatment.

In this concluding chapter I consider some factors that may help to account for diverging tendencies characterizing Jewish and Catholic approaches to bioethics. It should be kept in mind throughout that these are diverging tendencies between overlapping spectra, rather than sharp differences between monolithic approaches. I then review briefly the common ground between Jewish and Roman Catholic views and consider the significance of this convergence. Finally, I consider what Jewish and Roman Catholic approaches may learn from one another and the significance of these approaches for public policy in nations such as the United States.

Diverging Tendencies

Methodology: Telos and Duty

Jewish and Catholic thinkers alike attend to what might be characterized as teleological concerns (the end of the human person and society) and deontological concerns (specific duties and prohibitions). On the whole, Catholic theologians tend to give teleological analysis a more decisive role in ethical deliberations.[3] For many diverse Catholic thinkers, the patterns of nature and the appropriate ends of the human person can be known with a significant degree of precision and confidence. Ethical judgments tend to derive from these understandings of humans and the world. Jewish thinkers tend to be more modest in claims regarding knowledge of patterns and purposes and judge that ethical responsibilities may be known with greater precision and confidence. Although this theme is not universal, it can be found in sources ranging from the book of Exodus to Emmanuel Levinas's understanding of ethics as first philosophy.[4]

These divergent tendencies emerged over centuries of the development of the two traditions. They also accord with fundamental doctrinal understandings. For the Jewish tradition, God's fullest revelation, given in love, is represented by the Torah. At Mount Sinai the people of Israel heard God's words and committed themselves to fulfill God's *mitzvot* in a covenantal relationship. The call of Deuteronomy, "You shall love the Lord your God with all your heart and with all your soul and with all your might," is followed immediately by the corollary, "These words which I command you today shall be upon your heart," taught to children, spoken, and lived out in daily life. For developing rabbinic Judaism, study of God's word became a central means for encountering and worshiping God as well as for understanding God's will.[5]

In the Catholic and Christian tradition, God's most perfect revelation is Jesus Christ. The New Testament proclaims that in Jesus, God's word becomes flesh. "In this way the love of God was revealed to us: God sent his only Son into the world so that we might have life through him." Developing Christian tradition understands Jesus himself, rather than any sayings, as the foundational and true guide for humanity.[6] Catholic thinkers such as Ashley and O'Rourke connect their understanding of natural law and personalism to this revelation of the incarnate Son of God; the "historic model of true humanity is first of all Jesus the Christ."[7]

Although both elements may be found in Judaism and Catholicism alike, a Jewish inclination to mitzvah and a Catholic leaning to a teleological model have appeared throughout this book. In discussing euthanasia, Catholic thinkers on both sides of the issue utilize a model of a good death as a reference point. Even some of those who are opposed to euthanasia are reluctant to legally prohibit it for those who find such a death appropriate. Jewish writers more uniformly oppose legalizing euthanasia, perhaps in part because of the tradition's appreciation of the central role of law in shaping communal and personal life. Although overlapping spectra may be found regarding decisions at the end of life, on the whole Jewish writers are more likely to understand a duty to heal and preserve life to be decisive. Catholic writers are more likely to be confident in their identification of the *telos* or purpose of human life and to judge on that basis that some treatments should be forgone because they do not contribute to that purpose or that some lives need not be maintained because there is no possibility of fulfilling life's purpose.

The magisterium and many Catholic theologians oppose all uses of in vitro fertilization and other technologies that attempt to create children without respecting the appropriate pattern of procreation, as found in nature and willed by God. Even Catholic theologians who accept IVF try to reconcile it with a normative pattern linking marriage, sex, and procreation. Jewish thinkers are much more likely to frame the issue in terms of duties or *mitzvot*. Some argue against many uses of IVF to avoid violating specific prohibitions of the tradition. Others support uses of IVF by arguing that they would not violate prohibitions and positively emphasize the *mitzvot* of procreation, pursuing marital harmony, and relieving suffering. Finally, Catholic thinkers are more likely to insist on a single tier of access to health care and to accept rationing that denies needed treatment to some individuals, to strengthen the common good and build a morally better community. Jewish thinkers are more likely to support the right of individuals to pay for additional health care, in part because doing so fulfills the *mitzvot* of preserving health and saving life. Similarly, Jewish thinkers tend to oppose rationing because it would compromise the moral imperative to provide needed healing to persons in need, understood as a perfect duty.

Biological Teleology

Biological teleology, which is virtually absent from Jewish ethics, plays a significant and at times decisive role for Catholic moral theology. As I note in chapter 1, such concerns are common among Catholic thinkers historically, including Thomas Aquinas. Many contemporary thinkers argue that failure to respect intrinsic biological patterns (say, through artificial contraception or IVF) entails a failure to respect oneself as an embodied person, and hence constitutes an "intrinsically evil act" that can never be justified. Other thinkers, such as proportionalists, criticize such views as physicalism. Nevertheless, they generally would regard interference with biological patterns as an "ontic" or "premoral" evil that counts seriously against the acceptability of an action, even if the action could be justified by competing ethical considerations.[8]

Attention to biological patterns is most prominent in discussion of IVF. For the magisterium and some Catholic thinkers, attempts to circumvent the natural patterns of procreation simply are wrong. For others, such deviations from nature represent disvalues that count against IVF, but not always decisively so. Some thinkers who argue against the magisterium that IVF could be permissible—even if some in vitro embryos are discarded—appeal to biological patterns in support of this leniency, noting that naturally fertilized ova frequently fail to implant.

Active Partnership and Passive Servitude

As I note in the Introduction, each tradition includes both calls to human activity—reflecting a principle of human stewardship—and cautions to respect and avoid usurping God's sovereignty. Each tradition endorses appropriate human activity, including interventions in the natural order. On the whole, the impetus for human activity tends to be somewhat stronger among Jewish writers, the injunctions of reverent restraint stronger among Catholics. As with many of the characteristics considered in this book, in this area thinkers represent overlapping spectra, so that on most issues one can find relatively activist Catholic views and relatively cautious Jewish opinions.

The divergent tendencies correlate with differences in the root narratives or master stories of the two faiths. As Michael Goldberg observes, throughout the narrative of the book of Exodus human actions provide crucial contributions to the process of salvation. The Hebrew midwives save the boys whom Pharaoh has condemned; Moses's mother prepares a basket and places him on the river; Pharaoh's daughter sees the basket and saves the child's life; Moses hears God's call after he chooses to turn aside to investigate the burning bush. God actively enters the narrative only after the Israelites cry out, and God miraculously causes the plagues after Moses and Aaron perform specified actions. Before the tenth plague, God calls on the Israelites to slaughter a lamb and place blood on their doorposts, thereby enabling "the Israelites to become active participants in the work of achieving their salvation." Even at the Sea of Reeds, God requires Moses to lift his staff and tell the Israelites to proceed before God splits the sea. The exodus leads to the revelation at Mount Sinai, with Israel's acceptance of a covenant with responsibilities of action. The text presents a model of "joint enterprise." "In Exodus, whatever promised salvation is wrought by God is never worked by him alone but always in conjunction with and on condition of some complementary action by human beings."[9]

In the Gospel of Matthew, in contrast, God works salvation purely by grace, with no significant human action contributing to redemption. All humans fail to do what they should: Jews, Romans, even disciples. Three disciples repeatedly fall asleep soon after Jesus asks them to stay awake, because "the spirit is willing but the flesh is weak"; Peter denies Jesus three times "before the cock crows." Goldberg summarizes that "in the end . . . things manage to work out after all, not because of any human doings, but solely because of those of God."[10]

On numerous issues, Jewish thinkers tend to take a more activist stance than their Catholic counterparts. The contrast may be clearest with regard to IVF. The magisterium and some Catholic theologians warn against an attempt to dominate the process of procreation or intentionally to produce a child. Humans must accept their role as servants in the process, respecting God's plan that is manifest in nature and biology. A couple simply should accept the blessing of a child when it naturally occurs, supervening on the mutual self-giving of marital intercourse. Jewish thinkers more consistently encourage IVF as appropriate to an active human role in partnership with God. With regard to decisions near the end of life, there is some tendency for Jewish thinkers to support aggressive treatment and be more reluctant to let go and leave the patient in God's hands.

Healing

Healing and medicine represent prime examples of human activity and human intervention in the natural course of events. Both Judaism and Catholicism overwhelmingly support the practice of medicine and provision of healing when it is needed. Healing tends to represent a more powerful imperative—and to be more broadly construed—in the Jewish tradition. In cases near the end of life, Jewish writers are more likely than Catholic writers to call for provision of all effective medical care, even when the benefit appears uncertain or costs escalate. Jewish thinkers are less likely to support rationing, which compromises the commitment to provide patients with needed healing. They also do not advocate a single-tier system, which would prohibit patients from expending resources in pursuit of the mitzvah of healing and preservation of life. Jewish authors are more likely than their Catholic counterparts to understand infertility as a disease and the use of reproductive technologies to represent mandated healing. For the magisterium and some Catholic theologians, abortion would never be permitted, even (in a rare case) to save the life of the mother. Jewish views support abortion in such cases—in large part because of different understandings of the status of the fetus or unborn child, but also because of the power of the imperative to heal and save life. Even Jewish authorities who are most opposed to abortion insist that it must be performed when required to save the mother's life. Many Jewish thinkers construe therapeutic abortion broadly to include psychological health and protection against even remote threats.

Life in This World

Both Judaism and Catholicism accord great value to life in this world, appreciating it as a great and basic good. Jewish thinkers are somewhat more likely to find the value of life to be decisive, however, and Catholic thinkers to subordinate the value of life in this world to eternal salvation (although diverse views may be found in each tradition). Observers sometimes have claimed that Judaism is a "this-worldly" religion and Christianity "other-worldly." Although this claim is oversimplified, it does reflect an element of truth. For many Catholic theologians, the central narrative of Jesus's death and resurrection has relativized the life of this world. Life in this world clearly is subordinated to spiritual development and life eternal.[11] Although Jewish views on this subject are complex and varied, few Jewish theologians would put things quite that way. A typical Jewish understanding is that life in this world and life eternal represent two goods that are each basic and incommensurable, neither serving only instrumentally for the other. As expressed in the third-century Mishnah, "Better is one hour of repentance and good deeds in this world than all of life eternal in the world to come; and better is one hour of bliss in the world to come than all of life in this world."[12] A divergence in emphasis accorded to life in this world is evident in the founding narratives of each tradition. In the exodus God saves Israel from death and physical oppression, so that the Israelites could serve God in their lives in this world. For the New Testament, Jesus does not bring physical redemption but comes "to save his people from their sins" (Matthew 1:21).

At least at the margins, such an understanding of the value of this-worldly life would tend to support greater emphasis on preserving life. Although each tradition includes a range of views, Jewish authorities are more likely than Catholics to espouse a vitalist position, in which the imperative to preserve physical life is decisive.[13] Jewish thinkers who are more ready to forgo life-sustaining treatment tend to be even more cautious than their Catholic counterparts in doing so. Most Catholics would accept Pope Pius XII's view that extraordinary measures are not obligatory because "a more strict obligation would be too burdensome for most men and would render the attainment of the higher, more important good too difficult"; indeed, more aggressive measures are permitted to a person only "as long as he does not fail in some more serious duty."[14] As I note in chapter 4, many Jewish thinkers would be sympathetic to Pius's concern to avoid burdens. Few would be as ready to forgo life-sustaining treatment in the name of a "higher, more important good" or so worried that preserving life and health might interfere with a "more serious duty."

Even Jewish authorities who are most opposed to abortion mandate it when it is required to save the mother's life, in part because of the power of the imperative to save life. The imperative to save life reinforces the implications of the imperative to heal for access to health care and against rationing. Esteem for life in this world also offers some support for enabling the birth of new life when reproductive technologies are required.

The Holocaust

The imperative to save life has been reinforced for Jewish thinkers by a history that includes centuries of discrimination and mistreatment, including the experience in the twentieth century of the Holocaust. In the aftermath of mass killings of Jews and threats to their physical survival, Jewish theologians may lean more heavily toward maintaining life-sustaining treatment. The experience of the Holocaust may lead more directly to caution about the legalization of euthanasia. The practice of mass murder in Nazi Germany began with active killing of severely ill persons and built on earlier proposals advanced by leading physicians in the 1920s, before the Nazis took power. (These proposals were limited to patients who were incurably ill and mandated safeguards such as review panels.) The concept of "life unworthy of life," developed by well-intentioned thinkers, helped pave the way for Nazi genocide.[15] This history seems to influence Jewish thinkers to avoid speaking of life that need not be sustained because of the lack of capacity for pursuing life's purpose, or basing treatment decisions on the patient's quality of life (even with the care and caution expressed by Catholic theologians who use these terms).

Jewish thinkers also are influenced by demographic concerns resulting from the Holocaust and other factors. In the late 1930s there were about 16 million Jews in the world, representing about 0.85 percent of the total global population. About 6 million Jews were killed in the Holocaust. The current world Jewish population is about 13 million, which represents about 0.22 percent of the world's population. (For purposes of comparison, the world Catholic population was about 332 million in the late 1930s—17.9 percent of the total population—and now is about 1 billion, or 17.4 percent.)[16] The number of

Jews alive today is significantly smaller than the number alive before the Holocaust, even as the world population has tripled.

For at least some Jewish thinkers, these demographic concerns reinforce the tradition's value of procreation and children. David M. Feldman writes that "the historical circumstance of frequent massacres and forced conversions, with their decimation of Jewish communities, served to elicit compensatory tendencies. The people's will to replenish its depleted ranks gave an added dimension to its instinctive yearning for offspring."[17] Catholic thinkers today tend to be more concerned with overpopulation than underpopulation, providing some influence against the use of reproductive technologies, but influences could lead in the other direction if the demographics were different. Interestingly, Augustine suggests that a perceived demographic need for increased numbers could support a permissive judgment for less than ideal methods of reproduction. Although a life of celibacy generally is preferable to marriage and procreation, he argues, in the time of Abraham—when the physical survival of the community of Israel was at stake (to prepare for Christ, in accordance with God's plan)—procreation was a higher calling. Indeed, the need for procreation even justified polygamy in that time.

> There is not the need for procreation which there was then, when it was permissible for husbands who could have children to take other women for the sake of a more copious posterity, which certainly is not lawful now. The mysterious difference of times brings so great an opportunity of doing or of not doing something justly that, now, he does better who does not marry even one wife, unless he cannot control himself; then, however, they had without fault several wives, even they who could restrain themselves much more easily, except that piety in that time demanded something else.[18]

Sex and Family Life

The foregoing quotation from Augustine points to another difference in tendencies between Judaism and Roman Catholicism. Jewish and Catholic writers alike value family life and marital sexual relations. Both traditions historically have fostered some views that might be characterized as negative with respect to human sexuality. On the whole, however, Jewish views tend to be more affirming of family life in general and sex in particular. For Augustine—perhaps the central figure historically in the development of Christian views of sex—sexual activity is inextricably connected with concupiscence (lust and unruliness of the body associated with sin). Marital sexual intercourse is sinful unless undertaken to procreate or to support the spouse's fidelity. Although marriage is good, celibacy is better.[19] Over the centuries Catholicism has developed more positive views of sex, accepting unitive purposes of intercourse and the legitimacy of sexual pleasure. Nevertheless, historical suspicion of sexuality continues to exert some influence on some writers, and there remain some tendencies to regard celibacy as a higher good. Pope John Paul II writes that although marriage should be esteemed, "the church throughout her history has always defended the superiority of this charism [celibacy] to that of marriage, by reason of the wholly singular link which it has with the kingdom of God."[20]

Historically, Judaism consistently has understood marriage and children to be part of the ideal of human fulfillment, representing a religious responsibility. In contrast to the Catholic tradition, Jewish tradition has considered celibacy as—at best—the less perfect way. Sexual relations between husband and wife have been viewed positively, and sexual pleasure is legitimate. Indeed, marital sexual activity consistently has been considered a mitzvah, for purposes of companionship and pleasure even when procreation is not possible.[21] The prominence that Judaism gives to sexuality and family life also provides some general support to the use of reproductive technologies; an infertile couple is deprived of an important aspect of normal human fulfillment and accordingly should be helped to have a child.

Divergent approaches to sexuality also contributed to differing views of contraception. Catholic tradition has prohibited absolutely all artificial contraception—classically because contraception would repudiate the legitimizing purpose of procreation, more recently because contraception would separate the unitive and procreative aspects of the sexual act. Accordingly, Pope Pius XII proclaims that if pregnancy must be avoided (and "use of the sterile period" would not be effective), "there is but one way open, that of complete abstinence from every complete exercise of the natural faculty."[22] For traditional Jewish sources, abstinence not only would sacrifice the good of marital intercourse, it would preclude the fulfillment of a mitzvah. Although many Jewish sources generally prohibit artificial contraception, exceptions are made to avoid threats to the woman's health, while allowing marital intercourse to continue.[23] As I note in chapter 6, the magisterium and many Catholic theologians link the absolute prohibition of IVF to the absolute prohibition of artificial contraception. For Jewish thinkers, any linkage would tend to support the use of reproductive technologies when medically required.

As I note in chapter 5, differing approaches to contraception likely have exerted some influence on approaches to abortion. Historically, both traditions have strongly linked the prohibition against abortion to that against contraception. The Catholic absolute prohibition of contraception would cohere with an absolute prohibition of abortion. For Jewish authorities, the precedent of contraception would support a general prohibition of abortion, with exceptions to protect the woman's life and health. Although new arguments and considerations have developed over the centuries, for some authors the linkage between contraception and abortion persists, and traditional precedent generally exerts a powerful force in each tradition.

Points of Convergence

The considerations discussed in the preceding section are significant in explaining the divergences in tendencies between Jewish and Catholic approaches to bioethics. Yet one should not lose the forest for the trees. Jewish and Catholic views on these issues represent not opposed monolithic positions but overlapping spectra, reflecting many of the same basic values and concerns, in which a moral theologian in one faith community is likely to have more in common with some counterparts in the other community than with some thinkers in his or her own.

Jewish and Catholic writers share important common ground. Although important doctrinal beliefs separate the faith communities, with regard to practical ethical judgments the differences are much less stark. Overwhelmingly, Jewish and Catholic writers frame bioethical issues in similar ways, appeal to the same basic values, and raise similar concerns. The many ethical disputes surveyed in this book almost never take the form of Jewish thinkers as a group disagreeing with

Catholic thinkers as a group. Almost invariably, if an ethical judgment is supported by a strong consensus within one faith community, that consensus extends to much of the other faith community as well.

In addition to the shared basic values discussed in the introduction to this book, several additional points of consensus emerge. The inherent value and intrinsic dignity of all persons must be respected. Patients who are severely ill should receive adequate pain relief, as well as personal and spiritual support. Attention should be given to contemporary factors that tend to lead to abortion, including selfishness, poverty, and sexual irresponsibility. More should be done to support families and care for disabled persons. All members of society should be assured access to at least a basic level of health care. This common ground on particular judgments as well as basic values may reflect, in part, the formative influence of the values of the Hebrew Bible in both Judaism and Roman Catholicism, filtered through the different sacred writings and modes of reasoning developed in each tradition over the centuries.[24]

Many points of Jewish-Catholic consensus are shared widely beyond the two faith communities. One area in which religious writers as a group tend to differ from many others in bioethics concerns autonomy. Among the many arguments put forth by diverse writers, few explicitly present autonomy as an important value justifying a rule or policy. At the same time, most authors acknowledge a significant role for individual as well as communal choices in ethical decision making. In nations such as the United States, autonomy sometimes is discussed in black-and-white terms. For some writers, it seems at times as if a momentary preference of an atomistic individual should always be morally (not only legally) decisive, at least if the choice does not immediately and obviously impose tangible harm on identifiable individuals. For others, objective right and good readily can be determined in any situation, in a manner that is clear and unambiguous, and ideally that good would be imposed.

For most of the writers discussed in this book, matters are not that simple. More liberal as well as more conservative writers center their arguments on objective moral values, such as human well-being and respect for the intrinsic dignity of persons. As I note in chapter 4, few if any Jewish or Catholic writers justify forgoing life-sustaining treatment because of a right to die or simply because the patient should be able to do whatever he or she wants with his or her own life. A patient's decision generally should be respected because the patient is the best judge of when treatment is excessively burdensome or because God grants people significant authority as stewards over their lives, even though their lives are not fully their own. On the other hand, even the most vitalist of Orthodox Jewish authorities tend to allow some legitimate room for patient choice when a course of treatment involves significant risk, may not be effective, or has plausible alternatives. As several writers have noted, uncertainty represents the clinical norm; de facto, there is significant room for patient decisions.[25]

Similarly, as I note in chapter 5, few if any Jewish or Catholic writers simply advocate a prochoice view of abortion by claiming that the woman has an absolute right to determine what happens to her own body. Even the most liberal authors acknowledge that abortion entails significant moral costs and that individuals and society alike have the responsibility to act to diminish the likelihood of abortion. Writers accept women's choices of abortion not simply on the basis of autonomy but on the basis of claims regarding the woman's health and objective well-being. On the other hand, even writers who most forcefully argue that abortion would be objectively wrong in any situation generally acknowledge that there are some circumstances in which a woman's choice of abortion may be motivated by a desire to protect important values and may be blameless.[26]

Both Judaism and Catholicism traditionally have assumed a stance of ethical realism, in which some things really are good and others evil, some actions are objectively right and others wrong. Yet both traditions acknowledge that in the complexities of life it is not always obvious which course of action would reflect the right and the good. Individuals require practical reason in some form (conscience, discernment, prudence, judgment) to apply objective moral considerations to the particular situations and choices of their lives. They have some degree of authority and responsibility to formulate these individual judgments, specifying and building on the objective guidance of the tradition.[27]

Responding to Divergence and Convergence

The Mishnah reports that Ben Zoma, a second-century sage, taught, "Who is wise? The one who learns from every person" (*Avot* 4:1).

Jewish ethics and Catholic ethics have something to learn from all approaches to ethics. The interaction of Jewish and Catholic ethics can be particularly fruitful, however, because these traditions share fundamental values yet offer distinct perspectives on the implications of these (and other) values for the ethical life. In areas of divergence, members of each faith community may have much to learn from dialogue with the other. Historically these differences often have led to frustration and hostility. There also is benefit to be gained, however, by considering insights from a tradition that is both similar and distinctive. As Rabbi David Hartman has observed, a "religious culture has greater opportunities for inner purification and depth when it widens its range of perception through exposure to modes of thought and experiences that stem from other cultural frameworks."[28]

Dialogue with a tradition that differs from yet shares much with one's own could at least play a heuristic role, helping one to envision new possibilities or become sensitive to concerns that arise from shared values. To the extent that the two traditions have differing inclinations, they may complement each other. For example, both Judaism and Roman Catholicism support a stance that includes respect for divine sovereignty and the responsibility of active human stewardship. Thoughtful consideration of writings in the other tradition may help thinkers to remain conscious of both sides of the balance, reinforcing for a Catholic thinker the need for appropriate human action or for a Jewish thinker the need for limits. The thoughtful and moderate writings of Richard McCormick might lead a Jewish moderate thinker to greater sensitivity to the concerns raised by the use of donor gametes or to appreciation of the compatibility of decisions to forgo life-sustaining treatment in a broader range of cases with respect for and appreciation of the sanctity of life. Conversely, encounters with Jewish thinkers might lead a Catholic moderate to greater flexibility in IVF or caution in forgoing life-sustaining treatment.

As one example of mutual learning, Catholic theologian Lisa Sowle Cahill cites Rabbi David Novak's development of the traditional Jewish model that compares a fetus, when pregnancy endangers the mother's life, to a "pursuer." "Such analogies to assault serve simultaneously to protect the mother and the fetus. . . . The fetus is to be killed if and only if there exists the gravest reason, i.e., threat to the mother's life."[29] My own earliest thinking about life-sustaining treatment was influenced by Jewish authors and texts expressing the greatest reluctance to forgo such treatment. Passive euthanasia, though not as bad as active euthanasia, seemed similarly problematic in representing the choosing of death because life does not appear worthwhile. Such a decision would not sit well with Jewish ethics and commitments. My thinking on this issue was informed by Roman Catholic discussion of ordinary and extraordinary treatment, as well as Paul Ramsey's model of "only caring for the dying"—itself influenced by classical Catholic discourse. Treatments might be forgone not because death was sought but to pursue a course of care that would be more helpful to the patient, or to avoid the excessive burdens aggressive treatment would entail. As framed by Gerald Kelly the question is, "How much does God demand that I do in order to preserve this life which belongs to God and of which I am only a steward?"[30] This framing of the issue strikes me as fundamentally compatible with Jewish ethics, and it has enabled me to consider Jewish values and traditional texts in a new light.[31]

Elements within Catholic or Jewish ethics could be legitimate even when they diverge from norms in the other. As Stuart Hampshire argues, one cannot simply pick and choose elements of different cultures because they may be incompatible with each other and fail to support a coherent way of life; Hampshire terms this claim the "no-shopping principle."[32] Nevertheless, conscious consideration of the insights of differing ethical traditions can afford a perspective that leads to each tradition being challenged and enriched. Each tradition is likely to have its own areas of remarkable insight and its own blind spots. Exposure to the views of another tradition could make one aware of unstated and unexamined assumptions. In some cases, responses to this challenge of considering another tradition could lead to modification in one's own tradition or at least the way that the tradition is understood, articulated, and applied.[33] Even when a position from the other tradition is not fully convincing or not fully appropriated, it may lead to refinements. Even where no substantive changes occur, a thinker may be led to greater appreciation of the distinctive contribution of his or her own tradition—and perhaps greater epistemological modesty.

Consideration of another tradition can lead to an enriched understanding of one's own tradition not only on substantive issues but also with regard to methodology. I suggest in chapter 2 that significant parallels mark recent discussion in Catholic moral theology concerning natural law and in Jewish ethics concerning covenant. Consideration of the methodology of another tradition can help one take a step back from often intricate arguments within one's own tradition to gain a sense of the broader shape of the discussion.

I have suggested that Catholic ethics tends to incline to a teleological approach and Jewish ethics a more deontological orientation. In general these approaches exhibit complementary strengths and limitations. Teleology conveys a clear sense of the point of the enterprise and how more particular rules and judgments fit into a picture that makes sense. At the same time, its rich portrayal of a complex good may leave one without clear direction regarding which aspects of that good take priority, how competing considerations should be balanced, or which responsibilities have special urgency. Alternatively, teleology could lead to claims that anything falling short of the ideal is absolutely prohibited.[34] An approach that focuses on duties can give a clear sense of moral imperatives, while allowing discretion in the pursuit of the good within side constraints. Too narrow a focus on duties, however, can lead to a shallow legalism that loses the overall sense of the moral life. Both Catholic and Jewish ethics include attention to both the good and the right, with differing emphases. For a thinker in one tradition, consideration of views from the other tradition can help to maintain proper balance in a holistic ethical life.[35]

The two traditions also manifest complementary strengths in addressing individuals outside the faith tradition. Roman Catholic magisterial documents do so in a nuanced manner. For example, the Vatican "Declaration on Euthanasia" clearly delineates a variety of audiences that the document addresses. It presents considerations that "concern in the first place all those who place their faith and hope in Christ," but it also speaks to adherents of other religious faiths, as well as "people of good will" of diverse philosophical and ideological allegiance.[36] Natural law provides a clear framework for articulating ethical concerns that in principle are relevant for all humans. At times, however, authors may find it difficult to appreciate the unavoidable particularity of their own stance and the reasonableness of others reaching different conclusions. As Lisa Sowle Cahill observes, natural law thinkers should "recognize that Catholic natural law thinking, while aiming at the 'universal,' is worked out within a historically particular religious tradition: Christianity as Catholicism."[37]

The traditional Jewish approach of addressing ethical issues from the standpoint of Israel's covenantal relationship with God generally, and halakhah in particular, facilitates appreciation that other communities and faiths legitimately may reach differing conclusions. At the same time, this traditional stance poses challenges in explaining how the findings of Jewish ethics can be relevant or persuasive to persons outside the faith community. Jewish ethics must be able to speak in a way that is relevant to non-Jews for several reasons. First, there is benefit in discourse across differing traditions. Jewish ethics could be enriched by such discourse, and, conversely, Jewish ethics could contribute to Catholic ethics and other approaches. In addition, Judaism teaches that some ethical responsibilities are incumbent on all persons.[38]

A special consideration that has emerged in recent centuries reflects the fact that most Jews today live as citizens in nation-states that include diverse religious and secular traditions. Jewish ethics makes important claims on many issues that require the response of national society. One example is access to health care. As I note in chapter 7, according to Jewish ethics (as well as Catholic ethics) all members of the community must be provided with access to needed health care—at least a "decent minimum" that preserves life and meets other basic needs.[39] The scope of assuring access to needed care, however, exceeds the abilities of individuals or particular religious communities. According to Jewish ethics, then, national society has a responsibility to assure access to health care, and Jews who are members of such a society have the responsibility to promote such action when needed, as it is in the United States. The challenge for Jewish ethics—even more daunting in some ways than for Catholic ethics—is articulating a contribution that could be meaningful and persuasive for others in national (or international) society.

On issues such as access to health care, Roman Catholic and Jewish perspectives offer important contributions to ethical and policy deliberations in countries such as the United States. The United States has no established religion, and even nations with an established religion would be well advised not to bluntly impose rulings of a particular religious denomination on public society. Nevertheless, in the context of dialogue within a pluralistic society, views from religious perspectives have important contributions to make and are as legitimate as those emerging from any other particular point of view. Developments in philosophy as well as in society have led to an increased awareness that all moral reasoning occurs within a particular context and reflects a particular tradition. There is no available neutral space of "just plain ethics" that can be pursued in a purely objective manner, abstracting from all particular viewpoints such as Judaism or Roman Catholicism.[40] As Cahill observes, "No politician, philosopher, or 'humanist' marches into the contest armed only with the sharp sword of reason, stripped naked of the costume of any moral culture—however invisible he or she might wish that clothing to be." Public policy discourse on bioethical issues "is actually a meeting ground of the diverse moral traditions that make up our society." Religious and secular traditions contribute to this discourse, making distinctive contributions when they articulate shared commitments and when they offer differing perspectives.[41] Similarly, Noam Zohar argues that although morality seeks to be universal in scope, "no specific moral tradition can lay an exclusive claim to embodying a general human faculty of practical reason." Zohar advocates an approach of "procedural pluralism, which amounts simply to a willingness to concede our limitations. With respect to any moral problem, there may in principle be a 'truth of the matter,' but all we possess are various discrete attempts to get at the right answer." Accordingly, Zohar, like Cahill, emphasizes the importance of attending to "voices in dialogue."[42]

Shared Roman Catholic and Jewish understandings, such as the responsibility to assure access to at least a basic level of health care to all members of society, stake out important common ground.[43] This common ground could be part of an overlapping consensus across divergent world views. Societal responsibility to assure access to care, for example, could represent a "locus of certitude" that diverse individuals and groups could support, even if they provide differing rationales for this shared commitment.[44] As Cahill notes, writings developed within a given religious tradition may support ethical positions that could be justified on other secular or religious grounds. "Consensus in and about the public order is contingent not on genuine universality, but on intelligibility and persuasiveness within a community of communities."[45]

Such a consensus could be politically important in the development of governmental policy—thus supporting the feasibility of such a position. It certainly would represent a powerful articulation of the shared values and commitments of society. In addition, the consensus may have a deeper significance in supporting the belief that access to health care ought to be provided. In surveying the philosophical studies prepared for the President's Commission on Biomedical Ethics, Daniel Wikler finds significance in an overlapping consensus of various philosophical approaches. He notes that rival theories agree that "every person ought to be assured of access to some decent minimum of health care services" and argues,

> This conclusion cannot be said to have been "proved" by this collection of arguments, but the fact that a recommendation of universal access to (at least some) health care follows from such disparate sets of premises suggests that the recommendation is "insensitive" to choice of moral theory. Even if we do not know which moral theory is correct, then, and thus cannot provide a ground-level-up proof that all should have access to a minimum of health care, such a belief has been rendered reasonable and perhaps even compelling.[46]

The inclusion of Judaism and Roman Catholicism (as well as other religious traditions) in this consensus bolsters the claim that the recommendation is theory-insensitive and thus strengthens the warranted status of the belief that access to health care ought to be assured.[47]

In seeking to build an overlapping consensus on access to health care, as well as other issues in bioethics and ethics generally, it makes sense for Jewish and Catholic ethicists to look to one another as promising coalition partners. Commitments to values such as the need for responsible stewardship for the earth's resources, the intrinsic dignity of each human person, and love of neighbor have important implications for our lives and our society.[48] A dialogue between the traditions may lead not only to better understanding of the other but also to better understanding of the self and deeper appreciation of the moral task at hand. According to the Talmud, Rabbi Akiba asserted that learning is great because learning leads to doing (*Kiddushin* 40b). The hope of this book is that Jewish and Catholic ethics learn from one another and that this learning will foster working together for the common good and the improvement of the world.

Notes

1. For general discussion of the specification and balancing of moral norms, see Tom L. Beauchamp and James F. Childress, *Principles of Biomedical Ethics*, 5th ed. (New York: Oxford University Press, 2001), 15–21.

2. James M. Gustafson, *Protestant and Roman Catholic Ethics: Prospects for Rapprochement* (Chicago: University of Chicago Press, 1978), 30–31, 156.

3. See discussion in chapter 1, as well as Benedict M. Ashley and Kevin D. O'Rourke, *Health Care Ethics: A Theological Analysis*, 4th ed. (Washington, D.C.: Georgetown University Press, 1997), 156–66. Catholic approaches tend to be teleological in the sense of understanding the ends of the human person and human society to be foundational in ethical deliberation—not necessarily in the consequentialist sense often associated with this term. Similarly, I am characterizing Jewish views as deontological in the general sense of orientation to duties or responsibilities, not necessarily in an absolutist or Kantian sense.

4. Emmanuel Levinas, "Ethics as First Philosophy," in *The Levinas Reader*, ed. Seán Hand (Oxford: Blackwell, 1989), 75–87.

5. Exodus 19:1–8; 20; Deuteronomy 6:4–9; Louis Jacobs, *Jewish Values* (Hartford, Conn.: Hartmore House, 1960), 11–30; *Emet Ve-Emunah: Statement of Principles of Conservative Judaism* (New York: Jewish Theological Seminary of America, Rabbinical Assembly, United Synagogue of America, 1988), 53–55.

6. John 1:14, 1 John 4:9; *Catechism of the Catholic Church* (Mission Hills, Cal.: Benziger, 1994), nn. 430–483, pp. 108–121.

7. Ashley and O'Rourke, *Health Care Ethics*, 168.

8. These proportionalists would understand harms to human persons also to represent ontic evil—which also could be justified, although less readily so.

9. Exodus 1–20, esp. 1–3, 12, 14; Michael Goldberg, *Jews and Christians: Getting Our Stories Straight* (Nashville, Tenn.: Abingdon, 1985), 100, 214, and generally 25–131. Rabbinic midrash amplifies the need for human activity by relating that God did not split the sea until after one Israelite, Nahshon son of Aminadab, walked into it proactively (Talmud, *Sotah* 37a).

10. Matthew, esp. 26; Goldberg, *Jews and Christians*, 215, 135–212 generally. Goldberg finds the Gospel's ethos epitomized by the parable of weeds among the wheat, in which the householder rejects his servants' offer to gather the weeds. The householder tells them simply to wait until the time of the harvest. "As the parable tells it, the task of putting things right belongs to God and God alone. By contrast, in the Exodus narrative, God's acts of

rectifying the situation were again and again dependent on . . . corresponding human action. Yet in the parable of the weeds, the householder's servants are specifically told not to act, as though their activity would constitute a fundamental usurpation of the authority which is rightfully their master's, and even worse, botch the job to boot!" (Matthew 13:24–30, Goldberg, *Jews and Christians*, 162). The evidence from the parables is more ambiguous than that from the Passion, however. The parable of the talents (Matthew 25:14–30), for example, provides some support for human initiative and activity.

The greater hesitancy of Catholic writers to rely on human action correlates with Catholic understandings of human sinfulness and original sin. Similar views of personal sin—wrongful actions committed by individuals—are found in both Judaism and Roman Catholicism. Catholicism tends to have a greater sense of Sin as a powerful and pervasive force. Catholic doctrine teaches that all people are afflicted by original sin and cannot live morally without God's grace. See Charles E. Curran, *The Catholic Moral Tradition Today: A Synthesis* (Washington, D.C.: Georgetown University Press, 1999), 37–40; James P. Hanigan, *As I Have Loved You: The Challenge of Christian Ethics* (Mahwah, N.J.: Paulist, 1986), 101–17; *Catechism of the Catholic Church*, nn. 386–406, pp. 97–103. Judaism traditionally teaches that humans have both an inclination for good and an inclination for evil and that God has graciously granted humans free will and the ability to choose the good. From the standpoint of Catholic belief, Jewish views might seem to represent Pelagianism. From the standpoint of Jewish belief, Catholic views might seem to cast doubt on God's mercy and justice (though Catholic understandings of sin tend to be closer to Jewish thought than is some Protestant theology; see Gustafson, *Protestant and Roman Catholic Ethics*, 6–12). Moses Maimonides writes in his *Mishneh Torah*, "Free will is bestowed on every human being. If one desires to turn toward the good way and be righteous, he has the power to do so. If one wishes to turn toward the evil way and be wicked, he is at liberty to do so. . . . This means that the power is in your hands, and whatever a man desires to do among the things that human beings do, he can do, whether they are good or evil" ("Laws of Repentance" 5: 1, 3, in *A Maimonides Reader*, ed. Isadore Twersky [New York: Behrman House, 1972], 78–79). Although doctrinal differences regarding sin likely exert an indirect influence on authors in bioethics, Catholic writers in bioethics devote little explicit discussion to sin and its significance in moral reasoning. Curran observes (and criticizes) this phenomenon in Catholic moral theology generally.

11. See John Paul II, *Evangelium Vitae: The Gospel of Life* (Washington, D.C.: United States Catholic Conference, 1995), n. 47, p. 83; Richard A. McCormick, *Health and Medicine in the Catholic Tradition* (New York: Crossroad, 1987), 51–52; Ashley and O'Rourke, *Health Care Ethics*,

396–97; *Catechism of the Catholic Church*, nn. 1005–1020, pp. 262–66; Bernard Häring, *The Law of Christ*, vol. 1, trans. Edwin G. Kaiser (Westminster, Md.: Newman, 1963), 141–43.

12. Attributed to Rabbi Jacob, *Avot* 4:21.

13. As long as prohibitions against murder, idolatry, and adultery are not violated; see discussion in introduction.

14. Pope Pius XII, "The Prolongation of Life," *The Pope Speaks* 4 (1958): 395–96. See also the views developed from this statement by McCormick and others, in chapter 4.

15. Robert J. Lifton, *The Nazi Doctors: Medical Killing and the Psychology of Genocide* (New York: Basic Books, 1986), 14–15, 45–50; New York State Task Force on Life and the Law, *When Death Is Sought: Assisted Suicide and Euthanasia in the Medical Context* (New York: New York State Task Force on Life and the Law, 1994), 107.

16. *The Franciscan Almanac* (Paterson, N.J.: St. Anthony's Guild, 1938), 421; *American Jewish Year Book*, ed. David Singer and Lawrence Grossman (New York: American Jewish Committee, 2001), 538; Catholic Church, Rationarium Generale Ecclesiae, *Statistical Yearbook of the Church* (Vatican: Libreria Editrice Vaticana, 1999), 18. Estimates for the year 70 C.E. indicate a world Jewish population of about 8 million, out of a total population of 300 million, or 2.7 percent; see *Encyclopaedia Judaica*, s.v. "Population," 13: 871; *Encyclopaedia Britannica*, 15th ed. (1998), s.v. "Population," 25: 1041.

17. David M. Feldman, *Birth Control in Jewish Law*, rev. ed. (Northvale, N.J.: Jason Aronson, 1998), 51.

18. Augustine, "The Good of Marriage," chap. 15, trans. Charles T. Wilcox, in *The Fathers of the Church*, vol. 15, *Saint Augustine: Treatises on Marriage and Other Subjects*, ed. Roy J. Deferrari (New York: Fathers of the Church, 1955), 31. See generally chaps. 15–22.

19. Augustine, "The Good of Marriage," chaps. 6–7, 23; pp. 17, 44–45. See also David F. Kelly, "Sexuality and Concupiscence in Augustine," *Annual of the Society of Christian Ethics* (1983): 81–116.

20. John Paul II, *Familiaris Consortio: On the Family* (Washington, D.C.: United States Catholic Conference, 1982), n. 16, p. 14. See generally *Catechism of the Catholic Church*, nn. 2360–70, pp. 567–70; John T. Noonan, Jr., *Contraception: A History of Its Treatment by the Catholic Theologians and Canonists*, rev. ed. (Cambridge, Mass.: Belknap Press, Harvard University Press, 1986).

21. Traditionally, both husband and wife are expected regularly to engage in sexual intercourse, though either may decline in particular instances. Only the husband's responsibility is technically termed obligatory. This distinction may reflect the historical context of the Torah's proclamation

of conjugal rights in a polygamous culture (Exodus 21:10), or a sense that the wife's conjugal rights required greater legal protection than did the husband's (Feldman, *Birth Control in Jewish Law*, 21–105).

22. Pius XII, "The Apostolate of the Midwife," in *The Major Addresses of Pope Pius XII*, ed. Vincent A. Yzermans (St. Paul, Minn.: North Central Publishing Company, 1961), I: 170. The extensive Catholic debate on contraception is beyond the scope of this book.

23. Feldman, *Birth Control in Jewish Law*, 169–248, 297–304.

24. Arthur A. Cohen has argued against the existence of a "Judeo-Christian tradition," in part because of doctrinal differences regarding redemption and Jesus but also because Judaism and Christianity have lacked "the sharing of common concern and enterprise" that he considers requisite to a true tradition. He does acknowledge, however, significant "confluence" of doctrine. "Clearly it is not denied that both religions share compatible truths. There is a common sacred history; the ethical values to which appeal is made are similar; the eschatological vision overlaps; the normative institutions of both faiths are analogous. Christianity is, as Christians describe it, the younger brother to Judaism." Although Cohen emphasizes that Judaism and Christianity are distinct religions, he expresses confident hope in "Judeo-Christian fraternity": "Jews and Christians have joined together, during these past decades, not alone as men in their naked humanity but as men bearing psalms and seeing visions to oppose the evils of history and to work toward the conditions of peace" (*The Myth of the Judeo-Christian Tradition and Other Dissenting Essays* [New York: Schocken, 1971], iii, xii, 200, 220–21).

25. Avram Israel Reisner, "Care for the Terminally Ill: Halakhic Concepts and Values," in *Life and Death Responsibilities in Jewish Biomedical Ethics*, ed. Aaron L. Mackler (New York: Jewish Theological Seminary of America, Finkelstein Institute, 2000), 250–51; Benjamin Freedman, *Duty and Healing: Foundations of a Jewish Bioethic* (New York: Routledge, 1999), 163–70; J. David Bleich, "The Obligation to Heal in the Judaic Tradition: A Comparative Analysis," in *Jewish Bioethics*, ed. Fred Rosner and J. David Bleich (New York: Sanhedrin, 1979), 28–33.

26. John Paul II, *Evangelium Vitae*, n. 58, p. 105; Ashley and O'Rourke, *Health Care Ethics*, 257–59.

27. See discussion in chapters 1 and 2; *Catechism of the Catholic Church*, nn. 1776–1802, pp. 438–42; Hanigan, *As I Have Loved You*, 127–42; Aaron L. Mackler, "How Do I Decide? Practical Reason, Particular Judgments, and Holistic Concerns in Jewish Ethics," *Shofar* 18 (2000): 110–24.

28. David Hartman, *A Living Covenant: The Innovative Spirit in Traditional Judaism* (New York: Free Press, MacMillan, 1985), 103.

29. Lisa Sowle Cahill, "Abortion and Argument by Analogy," *Horizons* 9, no. 2 (1982): 277–78. Cahill notes (271) precedent for use of this model among Catholic theologians. See also chapter 6.

30. Paul Ramsey, *The Patient as Person* (New Haven, Conn.: Yale University Press, 1970), 113–64; Gerald Kelly, *Medico-Moral Problems* (St. Louis: Catholic Health Association, 1958), 132.

31. Moving beyond my own experience, similar developments have marked the growing acceptance among Jews of hospice over recent decades. Decades ago, Jewish ethics manifested suspicion at best regarding hospice. Hospice appeared to represent the choosing of death, instead of the courageous pursuit of life and healing Judaism demands. Most Jews have come to support hospice—influenced in part by Catholic and other Christian writings, as well as by the lived witness of hospice, molded decisively by Christian ethics. Considering the narrative of Jesus's death and the historical tradition of keeping company with the ill and dying, as well as Catholic reflections on the spiritual meaning of the dying process, it makes sense that Christians tended to accept modern hospice more readily than did Jews. Some differences between the faith communities persist. Nevertheless, Catholic and other Christian ethics can offer new insights and perspectives to enrich Jewish ethics.

32. Stuart Hampshire, *Morality and Conflict* (Cambridge, Mass.: Harvard University Press, 1983), 148. Hampshire argues for the essential differentiation of various ways of life in choosing among not fully compatible values. He allows that some norms, such as justice and utility, represent ethical criteria that hold across societies.

33. A commitment to reasoning within the context of a tradition and belief in the primacy of one's own tradition are compatible with modification of that tradition in response to outside input. See Alasdair MacIntyre, *After Virtue*, 2d ed. (Notre Dame, Ind.: University of Notre Dame Press, 1984), 270, 276; David Novak, *Jewish Social Ethics* (New York: Oxford University Press, 1992), 3–4.

34. As I note in chapter 1 and throughout this book, the first criticism has been made against proportionalists by more conservative theologians, the second against those theologians by proportionalists.

35. I have argued for the inclusion of varied and complementary elements in Jewish ethics in Aaron L. Mackler, "Cases and Principles in Jewish Bioethics: Toward a Holistic Model," in *Contemporary Jewish Ethics and Morality*, ed. Elliot N. Dorff and Louis E. Newman (New York: Oxford University Press, 1995), 177–93.

36. Congregation for the Doctrine of the Faith, "Declaration on Euthanasia," *Origins* 10 (1980): 155.

37. Lisa Sowle Cahill, "Can Theology Have a Role in 'Public' Bioethical Discourse?" *Hastings Center Report*, 20, no. 3 (1990, supp.): 13. A classical source supporting at least some degree of ethical pluralism is Thomas Aquinas, *Summa Theologiae* I-II 94, 4.

38. See chapter 2 and David Novak, *Natural Law in Judaism* (Cambridge: Cambridge University Press, 1998).

39. Individuals have primary responsibility to care for their own health and pay for needed care when they are able to do so. Contributions could be made by individual health care professionals and by organized religious communities.

40. See B. Andrew Lustig, "The Common Good in a Secular Society: The Relevance of a Roman Catholic Notion to the Healthcare Allocation Debate," *Journal of Medicine and Philosophy* 18 (1983): 569–71; Aaron L. Mackler, "Introduction," in Mackler, *Life and Death Responsibilities*, 5; and generally Jeffrey Stout, *Ethics After Babel: The Languages of Morals and Their Discontents* (Boston: Beacon, 1988).

41. Cahill, "Can Theology Have a Role," 13–14, 11.

42. Noam J. Zohar, *Alternatives in Jewish Bioethics* (Albany: State University of New York Press, 1997), 5. Zohar notes that intercultural dialogue requires "translation" between perspectives. "Forms of behavior, with their inherent potential for shaping our lives, serve as common currency. Addressed by both traditions, the same actions and ultimately the same character and biography are at stake. When a concrete problem is illuminated from different sources, it becomes a prism for mutual refraction. Hence the special relevance of an applied field like bioethics for intercultural dialogue" (11–12).

43. As I suggest in chapter 7, within this shared commitment the traditions have complementary perspectives. Jewish acceptance of differences in access to care (as long as all persons are guaranteed the basic minimum) may be more realistic, but Catholic advocacy of a single tier emphasizes values of equality and solidarity. Catholic acceptance of rationing may be more realistic, but Jewish opposition to rationing emphasizes the value of each individual person and the importance of healing.

44. See Albert R. Jonsen and Stephen Toulmin, *The Abuse of Casuistry: A History of Moral Reasoning* (Berkeley: University of California Press, 1988), 16–19.

45. Cahill, "Can Theology Have a Role," 13.

46. Daniel Wikler, "Philosophical Perspectives on Access to Health Care: An Introduction," in President's Commission for the Study of Ethical Problems in Medicine and Biomedical and Behavioral Research, *Securing Access to Health Care*, vol. 2 (Washington, D.C.: U.S. Government Printing Office, 1983), 48. Wikler's argument fits well with Norman Daniels's account of wide reflective equilibrium—in particular with Daniels's discussion of

intersubjective agreement and convergence as providing evidence of moral truth ("Wide Reflective Equilibrium and Theory Acceptance in Ethics," *Journal of Philosophy* 76 [1979]: 275–78). When the widening of reflective equilibrium by including the views of Judaism and Catholicism results in convergence with results obtained from other religious and secular approaches, it would seem that the evidence for moral truth is strengthened.

47. See similarly Aaron L. Mackler, "Judaism, Justice, and Access to Health Care," *Kennedy Institute of Ethics Journal* 1 (1991): 155.

48. See similarly Cahill, "Can Theology Have a Role," 12: "A person from a Jewish or Christian religious tradition might have sensibilities and interests that would make her or him more attuned to certain biblically based themes, such as the well-being of creation, God's providence, human responsibility, and human finitude and sinfulness. Other themes include love of neighbor and a 'preferential option for the poor' and vulnerable, mercy to others as God is merciful to us, forgiveness of others as we expect to be forgiven by God, and repentance for our sins. In nonreligious terms these themes cash out as service, not only autonomy; solidarity and integration within community; the dignity of all human beings, and special advocacy for the most vulnerable; sensitivity to our own finitude and the limits that we confront in all the projects we undertake."

Works Cited

Address, Richard F, ed. *A Time to Prepare*. Philadelphia: Union of American Hebrew Congregations, n.d.

American Fertility Society, Ethics Committee. "Ethical Considerations of Assisted Reproductive Technologies." *Fertility and Sterility* 62 (November 1994, suppl.).

American Jewish Year Book. Edited by David Singer and Lawrence Grossman. New York: American Jewish Committee, 2001.

Aquinas, Thomas. *Summa Theologiae*.

Arras, John D. "Toward an Ethic of Ambiguity." *Hastings Center Report* 14, no. 2 (1984): 25–33.

Ashley, Benedict M., and Kevin D. O'Rourke. *Health Care Ethics: A Theological Analysis*. 4th ed. Washington, D.C.: Georgetown University Press, 1997.

Auerbach, Shlomo. "Artificial Insemination." *Noam* 1 (1958): 145–66.

———. *Minhat Shlomo*. Jerusalem: Sha'arei Ziv Institute, 5746 (1985/86).

Augustine. "The Good of Marriage." In *Saint Augustine: Treatises on Marriage and Other Subjects*. Translated by Charles T. Wilcox. *The Fathers of the Church*, edited by Roy J. Deferrari, vol. 15. New York: Fathers of the Church, 1955.

Barry, Robert. "Feeding the Comatose and the Common Good in the Catholic Tradition." *Thomist* 53 (1989): 1–30.

Beauchamp, Tom L., and James F. Childress. *Principles of Biomedical Ethics*. 5th ed. New York: Oxford University Press, 2001.

Bernadin, Joseph. "Science and the Creation of Life." *Origins* 17 (1987): 21–26.

———. *The Consistent Ethic of Life*. Kansas City, Mo.: Sheed and Ward, 1988.

———. "The Consistent Ethic of Life and Health Care Reform." *Origins* 24 (1994): 60–64.

———. "Managing Managed Care." *Origins* 26 (1996): 21–26.

Bishops of Pennsylvania. "Nutrition and Hydration: Moral Considerations." *Origins* 21 (1992): 541–53.

Bleich, J. David. *Contemporary Halakhic Problems*, vol. 1. New York: Ktav and Yeshiva University Press, 1977.

———. *Judaism and Healing*. New York: Ktav, 1981.

———. *Contemporary Halakhic Problems*, vol. 4. New York: Ktav and Yeshiva University Press, 1995.

———. *Bioethical Dilemmas: A Jewish Perspective*. Hoboken, N.J.: Ktav, 1998.

Bleich, J. David, and Fred Rosner, eds. *Jewish Bioethics*. New York: San-hedrin, 1979.

Block, Richard Alan. "The Right to Do Wrong: Reform Judaism and Abor-tion." *Journal of Reform Judaism* 28, no. 2 (1981): 3–15.

Board of Rabbis of Southern California: Interfaith Committee, Los Angeles Chapter of the American Jewish Committee: Interreligious Affairs Com-mittee, and Roman Catholic Archdiocese of Los Angeles: Commission on Ecumenical and Interreligious Affairs. "Respect for Life: Jewish and Roman Catholic Reflections on Abortion and Related Issues." Los Ange-les, September 1977.

Borowitz, Eugene B. *Liberal Judaism*. New York: Union of American Hebrew Congregations, 1984.

———. *Exploring Jewish Ethics*. Detroit, Mich.: Wayne State University Press, 1990.

Boyle, Joseph M. "The Right to Health Care and its Limits." In *Scarce Med-ical Resources and Justice*, edited by Pope John XXIII Medical-Moral Research and Education Center, 13–25. Braintree, Mass.: Pope John XXIII Medical-Moral Research and Education Center, 1987.

Bresnahan, James F. "Observations on the Rejection of Physician-Assisted Suicide: A Roman Catholic Perspective." *Christian Bioethics* 1 (1995): 256–84.

Brickner, Balfour. "A Critique of Bleich on Abortion." *Sh'ma* 5, no. 85 (1975): 197–200.

Brody, Baruch A. "A Historical Introduction to Jewish Casuistry on Suicide and Euthanasia." In *Suicide and Euthanasia: Historical and Contempo-rary Themes*, edited by Baruch A. Brody, 39–75. Dordrecht, Nether-lands: Kluwer, 1989.

Cahill, Lisa Sowle. "Abortion and Argument by Analogy." *Horizons* 9, no. 2 (1982): 271–87.

———. "*In Vitro* Fertilization: Ethical Issues in Judaeo-Christian Perspec-tive." *Loyola Law Review* 32 (1986): 337–56.

———. "Notes on Moral Theology: Sanctity of Life, Quality of Life, and Social Justice." *Theological Studies* 48 (1987): 105–23.

———. "Abortion, Autonomy, and Community." In *Abortion and Catholicism: The American Debate*, edited by Patricia Beattie Jung and Thomas A. Shannon, 85–97. New York: Crossroad, 1988.

———. "Moral Traditions, Ethical Language, and Reproductive Technologies." *Journal of Medicine and Philosophy* 14 (1989): 497–522.

———. "Can Theology Have a Role in 'Public' Bioethical Discourse?" *Hastings Center Report* 20, no. 3, suppl. (1990): 10–14.

———. "Notes on Moral Theology: Bioethical Decisions to End Life." *Theological Studies* 52 (1991): 107–27.

———. "Abortion, Sex, and Gender: The Church's Public Voice." *America* 168, no. 18 (1993): 6–11.

———. "The Embryo and the Fetus: New Moral Contexts." *Theological Studies* 54 (1993): 124–42.

———. *Sex, Gender, and Christian Ethics*. Cambridge: Cambridge University Press, 1996.

———. "Good News and Bad." *Health Progress* 80, no. 4 (1999): 18–23.

Callahan, Sidney. "The Ethical Challenge of the New Reproductive Technology." In *Health Care Ethics: Critical Issues for the 21st Century*, edited by John F. Monagle and David C. Thomasma, 45–55. Gaithersburg, Md.: Aspen, 1998.

Canadian Royal Commission on New Reproductive Technologies. *Proceed with Care: Final Report of the Royal Commission on New Reproductive Technologies*. Ottawa: Royal Commission on New Reproductive Technologies, 1993.

Catholic Church. *Canons and Decrees of the Council of Trent*. Translated by H. J. Schroeder. St. Louis: B. Herder, 1941.

———. *The Documents of Vatican II*. Edited by Walter M. Abbott. New York: Corpus, 1966.

———. *Catechism of the Catholic Church*. Mission Hills, Cal.: Benziger, 1994.

———. *Vatican Council II: The Conciliar and Post Conciliar Documents*. New rev. ed. Edited by Austin Flannery. Northport, N.Y.: Costello, 1996.

Catholic Church, Congregation for the Doctrine of the Faith. "Declaration on Euthanasia." *Origins* 10 (1980): 154–57.

———. "Declaration on Procured Abortion." In *Vatican Council II: More Postconciliar Documents*, edited by Austin Flannery, 441–53. Collegeville, Minn.: Liturgical Press, 1982.

———. *Donum Vitae: Instruction on Respect for Human Life in Its Origin and on the Dignity of Procreation: Replies to Certain Questions of the Day*. Washington, D.C.: United States Catholic Conference, 1987.

242 · *Introduction to Jewish and Catholic Bioethics*

————. "Instruction on the Ecclesial Vocation of the Theologian." *Origins* 20 (1990): 117–26.

Catholic Church, International Theological Commission. "Memory and Reconciliation: The Church and the Faults of the Past." *Origins* 29 (2000): 625–44.

Catholic Church, Rationarium Generale Ecclesiae. *Statistical Yearbook of the Church*. Vatican: Libreria Editrice Vaticana, 1999.

Catholic Health Association of the United States. *With Justice for All? The Ethics of Healthcare Rationing*. St. Louis: Catholic Health Association of the United States, 1991.

Central Conference of American Rabbis (CCAR). "National Health Care." Resolution, June 1991. Available at www.ccarnet.org/cgi-bin/resodisp.pl?file=care&year=1991.

————. "In Vitro Fertilization and the Status of the Embryo." 1996/97. Available at www.ccarnet.org/cgi-bin/respdisp.pl?file=2&year=5757.

Cohen, Arthur A. *The Myth of the Judeo-Christian Tradition and Other Dissenting Essays*. New York: Schocken, 1971.

Condition of Jewish Belief, The. New York: Macmillan, 1966.

Conference of Reform Rabbis. "The Pittsburgh Platform." In *The Jew in the Modern World*, edited by Paul M. Mendes-Flohr and Jehuda Reinharz, 371–72. New York: Oxford University Press, 1980.

Connery, John. *Abortion: The Development of the Roman Catholic Perspective*. Chicago: Loyola University Press, 1977.

————. "Quality of Life." *Linacre Quarterly* 53 (1986): 26–33.

Curran, Charles E. *Contemporary Problems in Moral Theology*. Notre Dame, Ind.: Fides, 1970.

————. *Politics, Medicine, and Christian Ethics: A Dialogue with Paul Ramsey*. Philadelphia: Fortress, 1973.

————. *Ongoing Revision: Studies in Moral Theology*. Notre Dame, Ind.: Fides, 1975.

————. *New Perspectives in Moral Theology*. Notre Dame, Ind.: University of Notre Dame Press, 1976.

————. *Transition and Tradition in Moral Theology*. Notre Dame, Ind.: University of Notre Dame Press, 1979.

————. *The Catholic Moral Tradition Today: A Synthesis*. Washington, D.C.: Georgetown University Press, 1999.

Curran, Charles E., and Richard A. McCormick, eds. *Readings in Moral Theology, no. 8: Dialogue about Catholic Sexual Teaching*. Mahwah, N.J.: Paulist, 1993.

Daniels, Norman. "Wide Reflective Equilibrium and Theory Acceptance in Ethics." *Journal of Philosophy* 76 (1979): 256–82.

———. "Rationing Fairly: Programmatic Considerations." *Bioethics* 7 (1993): 224–33.

Davis, Henry. *Moral and Pastoral Theology*, vol. 1. New York: Sheed and Ward, 1935.

DeBlois, Jean, and Kevin D. O'Rourke. "Issues at the End of Life." *Health Progress* 76, no. 6 (1995): 24–27.

Dorff, Elliot N. *Conservative Judaism: Our Ancestors to Our Descendants.* Rev. ed. New York: United Synagogue of Conservative Judaism, 1996.

———, *Matters of Life and Death: A Jewish Approach to Modern Medical Ethics*. Philadelphia: Jewish Publication Society, 1998.

Dorff, Elliot N., and Louis E. Newman, eds. *Contemporary Jewish Ethics and Morality: A Reader*. New York: Oxford University Press, 1995.

Dougherty, Charles J. *Back to Reform: Values, Markets and the Health Care System*. New York: Oxford University Press, 1996.

Eisenberg, Daniel. "Is Managed Care Unethical?" *Maimonides* 3, no. 2 (1997): 3.

Eliyahu, Mordecai. "Destroying Fertilized Eggs and Fetal Reduction." *Tehumin* 11 (1991): 272–74.

Emet Ve-Emunah: Statement of Principles of Conservative Judaism. New York: Jewish Theological Seminary of America, Rabbinical Assembly, United Synagogue of America, 1988.

Encyclopaedia Judaica. 16 vols. Jerusalem: Keter, 1972.

Farley, Margaret. "Issues in Contemporary Christian Ethics: The Choice of Death in a Medical Context." Speech at Santa Clara University, May 1, 1995. Published as *The Santa Clara Lectures* 1, no. 3. Santa Clara, Calif.: Santa Clara University, 1995.

Feinstein, Moshe. *Iggerot Moshe*. 8 vols. New York: Moriah, 1959–96.

Feldman, David M. *Health and Medicine in the Jewish Tradition*. New York: Crossroad, 1986.

———. *Birth Control in Jewish Law*. Rev. ed. Northvale, N.J.: Jason Aronson, 1998.

Feldman, David M., and Fred Rosner, eds. *Compendium on Medical Ethics*. 6th ed. New York: Federation of Jewish Philanthropies of New York, 1984.

Finkelstein, Louis. "Human Equality in the Jewish Tradition." In *Aspects of Equality*, edited by Lyman Bryson, Clarence H. Faust, Louis Finkelstein, and R. M. MacIver, 179–205. New York: Harper and Brothers, 1956.

Fox, Marvin, ed. *Modern Jewish Ethics: Theory and Practice*. Columbus: Ohio State University Press, 1975.

Franciscan Almanac. Paterson, N.J.: St. Anthony's Guild, 1938.

Freedman, Benjamin. *Duty and Healing: Foundations of a Jewish Bioethic.* New York: Routledge, 1999.

Füchs, Josef. *Natural Law: A Theological Investigation.* Translated by Helmut Reckter and John A. Dowling. New York: Sheed and Ward, 1965.

Gillman, Neil. *Sacred Fragments: Recovering Theology for the Modern Jew.* Philadelphia: Jewish Publication Society, 1990.

———. *The Death of Death: Resurrection and Immortality in Jewish Thought.* Woodstock, Vt.: Jewish Lights, 1997.

Goldberg, Michael. *Jews and Christians: Getting Our Stories Straight.* Nashville, Tenn.: Abingdon, 1985.

Golding, Martin P. "Preventive vs. Curative Medicine: Perspectives of the Jewish Legal Tradition." *Journal of Medicine and Philosophy* 8 (1983): 269–86.

Grazi, Richard V., and Joel B. Wolowelsky. "Donor Gametes for Assisted Reproduction in Contemporary Jewish Law and Ethics." *Assisted Reproductive Reviews* 2 (1992): 154–60.

Grazi, Richard V., Joel B. Wolowelsky, and Raphael Jewelewicz. "Assisted Reproduction in Contemporary Jewish Law and Ethics." *Gynecological and Obstetric Investigations* 37 (1994): 217–25.

Greenberg, Blu. "Abortion: A Challenge to Halakhah." *Judaism* 25 (1976): 201–8.

Greenberg, Simon. *A Jewish Philosophy and Pattern of Life.* New York: Jewish Theological Seminary of America, 1981.

Grisez, Germain G. *Abortion: The Myths, the Realities, and the Arguments.* New York: Corpus, 1970.

Gudorf, Christine. "Making Distinctions." *Christianity and Crisis* 46 (1986): 242–44.

Gustafson, James M. *Protestant and Roman Catholic Ethics: Prospects for Rapprochement.* Chicago: University of Chicago Press, 1978.

Halevi, Hayyim David. "Disconnecting a Patient with No Prospect of Survival from a Respirator." *Tehumin* 2 (5741 [1980/81]): 297–305.

———. "On Fetal Reduction and the Halakhic Status of In Vitro Embryos." *Assia,* no. 47–48 (1990): 14–17.

Hampshire, Stuart. *Morality and Conflict.* Cambridge, Mass.: Harvard University Press, 1983.

Hanigan, James P. *As I Have Loved You: The Challenge of Christian Ethics.* Mahwah, N.J.: Paulist, 1986.

Häring, Bernard. *The Law of Christ,* vol. 1. Translated by Edwin G. Kaiser. Westminster, Md.: Newman, 1963.

———. *Medical Ethics.* Edited by Gabrielle L. Jean. Notre Dame, Ind.: Fides, 1973.

Harris, Jay M. *How Do We Know This? Midrash and the Fragmentation of Modern Judaism*. Albany: State University of New York Press, 1995.

Hartman, David. *A Living Covenant: The Innovative Spirit in Traditional Judaism*. New York: Free Press, Macmillan, 1985.

Herberg, Will. *Judaism and Modern Man: An Interpretation of Jewish Religion*. New York: Farrar Straus and Young, 1951; reprint, Atheneum, 1970.

Herring, Basil F. *Jewish Ethics and Halakhah for Our Time*. New York: Ktav and Yeshiva University Press, 1984.

Heschel, Abraham Joshua. *God in Search of Man: A Philosophy of Judaism*. New York: Farrar, Straus and Giroux, 1955.

Holy Letter. Translated by Seymour J. Cohen. Northvale, N.J.: Jason Aronson, 1993; reprint of New York: Ktav, 1976.

Israel Ministry of Health. Report of Steinberg Commission on the Care of the Terminally Ill Patient, 2002. Available (in Hebrew only) at www.health.gov.il/pages/default.asp?PageId=632&parentId=10&catId=6&maincat=1.

Jacob, Walter, ed. *American Reform Responsa*. New York: Central Conference of American Rabbis, 1983.

———. *Contemporary American Reform Responsa*. New York: Central Conference of American Rabbis, 1987.

———. *Questions and Reform Jewish Answers*. New York: Central Conference of American Rabbis, 1992.

Jacob, Walter, and Moshe Zemer, eds. *Death and Euthanasia in Jewish Law: Essays and Responsa*. Pittsburgh: Rodef Shalom Press, 1995.

———. *The Fetus and Fertility in Jewish Law: Essays and Responsa*. Pittsburgh: Rodef Shalom Press, 1995.

Jacobs, Louis. *Jewish Values*. Hartford, Conn.: Hartmore House, 1960.

Jakobovits, Immanuel. "Whether It Is Permitted to Hasten the Death of a Terminally Ill Patient Who Is Suffering." *Hapardes* 31, no. 1 (1956): 28–31; no. 3 (1956): 16–19.

———. "Jewish Views on Abortion." In *Abortion and the Law*, edited by David T. Smith, 12–43. Cleveland: Western Reserve University Press, 1967.

———. *Jewish Medical Ethics*. Rev. ed. New York: Bloch, 1975.

Jakobovits, Yoel. "Male Infertility: Halakhic Issues in Investigation and Management." *Tradition* 27, no. 2 (1993): 4–21.

Janssens, Louis. "Artificial Insemination: Ethical Considerations." *Louvain Studies* 7 (1980): 3–29.

John XXIII. *Pacem in Terris: Peace on Earth*. Washington, D.C.: National Catholic Welfare Conference, 1963.

John Paul II. *Laborem Exercens: On Human Work*. Washington, D.C.: United States Catholic Conference, 1981.

———. *Familiaris Consortio: On the Family*. Washington, D.C.: United States Catholic Conference, 1982.

———. *Veritatis Splendor: The Splendor of Truth*. Washington, D.C.: United States Catholic Conference, 1993.

———. *Evangelium Vitae: The Gospel of Life*. Washington, D.C.: United States Catholic Conference, 1995.

———. "Service Requesting Pardon." *Origins* 29 (2000): 645–48.

Jonsen, Albert R., and Stephen Toulmin. *The Abuse of Casuistry: A History of Moral Reasoning*. Berkeley: University of California Press, 1988.

Karo, Joseph. *Shulḥan Arukh*.

Keane, Philip S. *Health Care Reform: A Catholic View*. New York: Paulist, 1993.

Keenan, James F., and Myles Sheehan. "Life Supports: Sorting Bishops' Views." *Church* (winter 1992): 10–17.

Kellner, Menachem Marc, ed. *Contemporary Jewish Ethics*. New York: Sanhedrin, 1978.

Kelly, David F. *The Emergence of Roman Catholic Medical Ethics in North America*. New York: Edward Mellen Press, 1979.

———. "Sexuality and Concupiscence in Augustine." *Annual of the Society of Christian Ethics* (1983): 81–116.

———. *A Theological Basis for Health Care and Health Care Ethics*. Milwaukee, Wisc.: National Association of Catholic Chaplains, 1985.

———. *Critical Care Ethics: Treatment Decisions in American Hospitals*. Kansas City, Mo.: Sheed and Ward, 1991.

Kelly, Gerald. *Medico-Moral Problems*. St. Louis: Catholic Health Association, 1958.

Knauer, Peter. "The Hermeneutic Function of the Principle of Double Effect." In *Readings in Moral Theology, no. 1: Moral Norms and Catholic Tradition*, edited by Charles E. Curran and Richard A. McCormick, 1–39. New York: Paulist, 1979.

Kogan, Barry S., ed. *A Time to Be Born and a Time to Die: The Ethics of Choice*. New York: Aldine de Gruyter, 1991.

Human Sexuality: New Directions in American Catholic Thought: A Study Commissioned by the Catholic Theological Society of America. New York: Paulist, 1977.

Lauritzen, Paul. "Pursuing Parenthood: Reflections on Donor Insemination." *Second Opinion* 17, no. 1 (1991): 57–76.

———. *Pursuing Parenthood: Ethical Issues in Assisted Reproduction*. Bloomington: Indiana University Press, 1993.

Levinas, Emmanuel. "Ethics as First Philosophy." In *The Levinas Reader*, edited by Seán Hand, 75–87. Oxford: Blackwell, 1989.

Lifton, Robert J. *The Nazi Doctors: Medical Killing and the Psychology of Genocide*. New York: Basic Books, 1986.

Lustig, B. Andrew. "The Common Good in a Secular Society: The Relevance of a Roman Catholic Notion to the Healthcare Allocation Debate." *Journal of Medicine and Philosophy* 18 (1993): 569–87.

———. "Reform and Rationing: Reflections on Health Care in Light of Catholic Social Teaching." In *Secular Bioethics in Theological Perspective*, edited by Earl E. Shelp, 31–50. Dordrecht, Netherlands: Kluwer, 1996.

MacIntyre, Alasdair. *After Virtue*. 2d ed. Notre Dame, Ind.: University of Notre Dame Press, 1984.

Mackler, Aaron L. "Judaism, Justice, and Access to Health Care." *Kennedy Institute of Ethics Journal* 1 (1991): 143–61.

———. "How Do I Decide? Practical Reason, Particular Judgments, and Holistic Concerns in Jewish Ethics." *Shofar* 18 (2000): 110–24.

———. "Jewish and Roman Catholic Approaches to Bioethics: Convergence and Divergence in Method and Substance." *Louvain Studies* 25 (2000): 3–22.

Mackler, Aaron L., ed. *Life and Death Responsibilities in Jewish Biomedical Ethics*. New York: Finkelstein Institute and Jewish Theological Seminary of America, 2000.

Maguire, Daniel C. "The Freedom to Die." *Commonweal* 96 (1972): 423–27.

———. "A Catholic View of Mercy Killing." In *Beneficent Euthanasia*, edited by Marvin Kohl, 34–43. Buffalo, N.Y.: Prometheus, 1975.

Maguire, Daniel C., and James Tunstead Burtchaell. "The Catholic Legacy and Abortion: A Debate." *Commonweal* 114 (1987): 657–80.

Mahoney, John. *Bioethics and Belief: Religion and Medicine in Dialogue*. London: Sheed and Ward, 1984.

———. *The Making of Moral Theology: A Study of the Roman Catholic Tradition*. New York: Clarendon Press, Oxford University Press, 1987.

Maimonides, Moses. *Mishneh Torah*.

———. *The Guide of the Perplexed*. Translated by Shlomo Pines. Chicago: University of Chicago Press, 1963.

———. *A Maimonides Reader*. Edited by Isadore Twersky. New York: Behrman House, 1972.

May, William E., Robert Barry, et al. "Feeding and Hydrating the Permanently Unconscious and Other Vulnerable Persons." *Issues in Law and Medicine* 3, no. 3 (1987): 203–17.

McCartney, James J. "The Right to Die: Perspectives from the Catholic and Jewish Traditions." In *To Die or Not to Die? Cross-Disciplinary*,

Cultural, and Legal Perspectives on the Right to Choose Death, edited by Arthur S. Berger and Joyce Berger, 13–24. New York: Praeger, 1990.

McCormick, Richard A. "Human Significance and Christian Significance." In *Norm and Context in Christian Ethics*, edited by Gene H. Outka and Paul Ramsey, 233–61. New York: Charles Scribner's Sons, 1968.

———. "Notes on Moral Theology: The Abortion Dossier." *Theological Studies* 35 (1974): 312–59.

———. *How Brave a New World?* Washington, D.C.: Georgetown University Press, 1981.

———. *Notes on Moral Theology 1965–1980*. Washington, D.C.: University Press of America, 1981.

———. *Health and Medicine in the Catholic Tradition*. New York: Crossroad, 1984.

———. "Therapy or Tampering? The Ethics of Reproductive Technology." *America* 153 (1985): 396–403.

———. *The Critical Calling: Reflections on Moral Dilemmas Since Vatican II*. Washington, D.C.: Georgetown University Press, 1989.

———. "Who or What Is the Preembryo?" *Kennedy Institute of Ethics Journal* 1 (1991): 1–15.

———. "Some Early Reactions to *Veritatis Splendor*." *Theological Studies* 55 (1994): 481–506.

———. "Technology, the Consistent Ethic, and Assisted Suicide." *Origins* 25 (1995): 459–64.

———. "A Catholic Perspective on Access to Care." *Cambridge Quarterly of Healthcare Ethics* 7 (1998): 254–59.

Meier, Levi, ed. *Jewish Values in Bioethics*. New York: Human Sciences Press, 1986.

Montefiore, C. G., and H. Loewe, eds. *A Rabbinic Anthology*. New York: Schocken, 1974.

National Conference of Catholic Bishops. "Pastoral Letter on Health and Health Care." *Origins* 11 (1981): 396–402.

———. *The Challenge of Peace: God's Promise and Our Response*. Washington, D.C.: United States Catholic Conference, 1983.

———. *Economic Justice for All: Pastoral Letter on Catholic Social Teaching and the U.S. Economy*. Washington, D.C.: United States Catholic Conference, 1986.

———. "Criteria for Evaluating Health Care Reform." *Origins* 22 (1992): 23–24.

———. "Resolution on Health Care Reform." *Origins* 23 (1993): 98–102.

————. "Ethical and Religious Directives for Catholic Health Care Services." *Origins* 24 (1994): 449–64.

National Conference of Catholic Bishops Committee for Pro-Life Activities. "Nutrition and Hydration: Moral and Pastoral Reflections." *Origins* 21 (1992): 705–12.

Nebenzal, Avigdor. "In Vitro Fertilization: Notes." *Assia*, no. 35 (1983): 5.

Neusner, Jacob. "Was Rabbinic Judaism Really 'Ethnic'?" *Catholic Biblical Quarterly* 57 (1995): 281–305.

New American Bible with Revised New Testament (NAB). Washington, D.C.: Confraternity of Christian Doctrine, 1986.

New Jersey Catholic Conference. "Providing Food and Fluids to Severely Brain Damaged Patients." *Origins* 16 (1987): 582–84.

New York State Task Force on Life and the Law. *When Death Is Sought: Assisted Suicide and Euthanasia in the Medical Context.* New York: New York State Task Force on Life and the Law, 1994.

————. *Assisted Reproductive Technologies: Analysis and Recommendations for Public Policy.* New York: New York State Task Force on Life and the Law, 1998.

Newman, Louis E. *Past Imperatives: Studies in the History and Theory of Jewish Ethics.* Albany: State University of New York Press, 1998.

Noonan, John T., Jr. *Contraception: A History of Its Treatment by the Catholic Theologians and Canonists.* Rev. ed. Cambridge, Mass.: Belknap Press, Harvard University Press, 1986.

————. "Development in Moral Doctrine." *Theological Studies* 54 (1993): 662–77.

Noonan, John T., Jr., ed. *The Morality of Abortion: Legal and Historical Perspectives.* Cambridge, Mass.: Harvard University Press, 1970.

Novak, David. *Law and Theology in Judaism.* New York: Ktav, 1974.

————. "Bioethics and the Contemporary Jewish Community." *Hastings Center Report* 20, 3, suppl. (1990): 14–17.

————. *Jewish Social Ethics.* New York: Oxford University Press, 1992.

————. *Natural Law in Judaism.* Cambridge: Cambridge University Press, 1998.

O'Connell, Timothy E. *Principles for a Catholic Morality.* Rev. ed. New York: HarperSanFrancisco, HarperCollins, 1990.

Oregon and Washington Bishops. "Living and Dying Well." *Origins* 21 (1991): 345–52.

O'Rourke, Kevin. "Evolution of Church Teaching on Prolonging Life." *Health Progress* 69, no. 1 (1988): 28–35.

Paris, John J. "Autonomy and Physician-Assisted Suicide." *America* 176, no. 17 (1997): 11–14.

Pellegrino, Edmund D., and Alan I. Faden, eds. *Jewish and Catholic Bioethics: An Ecumenical Dialogue*. Washington, D.C.: Georgetown University Press, 1999.

Pellegrino, Edmund D., John Collins Harvey, and John P. Langan, eds. *Gift of Life: Catholic Scholars Respond to the Vatican Instruction*. Washington, D.C.: Georgetown University Press, 1990.

Pius XI. *Casti Connubii: On Christian Marriage*. New York: Barry Vail, 1931.

Pius XII. *Humani Generis*. New York: Paulist, 1950.

———. "Marriage and Parenthood." *The Pope Speaks* 3 (1956): 191–97.

———. "The Prolongation of Life." *The Pope Speaks* 4 (1958): 393–98.

———. "The Apostolate of the Midwife." In *The Major Addresses of Pope Pius XII*, edited by Vincent A. Yzermans, vol. 1, 160–76. St. Paul, Minn.: North Central Publishing Co., 1961.

Plaut, W. Gunther, and Mark Washofsky, eds. *Teshuvot for the Nineties: Reform Judaism's Answers to Today's Dilemmas*. New York: Central Conference of American Rabbis, 1997.

Rabbinical Council of America. *Appointment of a Health Care Agent/Advance Directive*. New York: Rabbinical Council of America, n.d.

Rabinowitz, Gedaliah Aharon, and Mordecai Koenigsberg. "The Definition of Death and Determination of Its Time according to Halakhah." *Hadarom* no. 32 (1970): 59–76.

Rahner, Karl. *The Love of Jesus and the Love of Neighbor*. Translated by Robert Barr. New York: Crossroad, 1983.

Ramsey, Paul. *The Patient as Person*. New Haven, Conn.: Yale University Press, 1970.

Reich, Warren T., ed. *Encyclopedia of Bioethics*. 2d ed. 5 vols. New York: Simon and Schuster Macmillan, 1995.

Reines, Alvin J. "Reform Judaism, Bioethics, and Abortion." *Journal of Reform Judaism* 37, no. 1 (1990): 43–59.

Rosner, Fred. "Managed Care: A Contradiction or Fulfillment of Jewish Law?" n.d. ftp://ftp.ijme.org/pub/Transcripts/Rosner/rmanagedcare.txt (accessed April 16, 1998; no longer available).

———. *Modern Medicine and Jewish Ethics*. 2d ed. Hoboken, N.J.: Ktav, 1991.

Roth, Joel. *The Halakhic Process: A Systemic Analysis*. New York: Jewish Theological Seminary of America, 1986.

Schechter, Solomon. "Introduction to Studies in Judaism: First Series." In *Studies in Judaism: A Selection*. Philadelphia: Jewish Publication Society, 1958.

Shannon, Thomas A., and Allan B. Wolter. "Reflections on the Moral Status of the Pre-embryo." *Theological Studies* 51 (1990): 603–26.

Siegel, Seymour, ed. *Conservative Judaism and Jewish Law.* New York: Rabbinical Assembly, 1977.

Smith, Russell E., ed. *Concerning Human Life.* Braintree, Mass.: Pope John XXIII Medical-Moral Research and Education Center, 1989.

Soloveitchik, Hayim. *Hiddushei R. Hayim Halevi al HaRambam.* Israel: n.p., 1992.

Steinberg, Avraham. *Encyclopedia of Jewish Medical Ethics.* 6 vols. Jerusalem: Schlesinger Institute, 1988–98.

Sternbuch, Moshe. "Test-Tube Baby." *Bishvilei Harefu'ah* 8 (5747/1987): 29–36.

Stout, Jeffrey. *Ethics After Babel.* Boston: Beacon, 1988.

Sullivan, Francis A. *Magisterium: Teaching Authority in the Catholic Church.* New York: Paulist, 1983.

Tanakh: A New Translation of the Holy Scriptures according to the Traditional Hebrew Text (NJPS). Philadelphia: Jewish Publication Society, 1985.

Tendler, Moshe D., and Fred Rosner. "Quality and Sanctity of Life in the Talmud and the Midrash." *Tradition* 28, no. 1 (1993): 18–27.

Texas Bishops. "On Withholding Artificial Nutrition and Hydration." *Origins* 20 (1990): 53–55.

Tuchinski, Yehiel M. *Gesher Hahayyim.* Jerusalem: Solomon, 1960.

Tucker, Gordon. "God, the Good, and Halakhah." *Judaism* 38 (1989): 365–76.

Tuohey, John F. "The Implications of the *Ethical and Religious Directives for Catholic Health Care Services* on the Clinical Practice of Resolving Ectopic Pregnancies." *Louvain Studies* 20 (1995): 41–57.

Unterman, Issar. "On the Matter of Saving of the Life of a Fetus." *Noam* 6 (1963): 1–11.

Uziel, Ben Zion. *Mishpetei Uziel.* Jerusalem: Va'ad L'hotza'at Kitvei Harav, 1995.

Vacek, Edward V. "Notes on Moral Theology: Vatican Instruction on Reproductive Technology." *Theological Studies* 49 (1988): 110–31.

Waldenberg, Eliezer Yehudah. *Tzitz Eliezer.* 2d ed. 15 vols. Jerusalem: n.p., 1985.

Wallace, Marilyn, and Thomas W. Hilgers, eds. *The Gift of Life: The Proceedings of a National Conference on the Vatican Instruction on Reproductive Ethics and Technology.* Omaha, Neb.: Pope Paul VI Institute Press, 1990.

Walter, James J. "The Meaning and Validity of Quality of Life Judgments in Contemporary Roman Catholic Medical Ethics." *Louvain Studies* 13 (1988): 195–208.

Waxman, Mordecai, ed. *Tradition and Change: The Development of Conservative Judaism*. New York: Rabbinical Assembly, 1958.

Wikler, Daniel. "Philosophical Perspectives on Access to Health Care: An Introduction." In President's Commission for the Study of Ethical Problems in Medicine and Biomedical and Behavioral Research, *Securing Access to Health Care*, vol. 2, 109–51. Washington, D.C.: U.S. Government Printing Office, 1983.

———. "Ethics and Rationing: 'Whether,' 'How,' or 'How Much'?" *Journal of the American Geriatrics Society* 40 (1992): 398–403.

Wildes, Kevin W. "Ordinary and Extraordinary Means and the Quality of Life." *Theological Studies* 57 (1996): 500–12.

Wildes, Kevin W., ed. *Infertility: A Crossroad of Faith, Medicine and Technology*. Dordrecht, Netherlands: Kluwer, 1997.

Zohar, Noam J. *Alternatives in Jewish Bioethics*. Albany: State University of New York Press, 1997.

Zoloth, Laurie. "Face to Face, Not Eye to Eye: Further Conversations on Jewish Medical Ethics." *Journal of Clinical Ethics* 6 (1995): 222–31.

———. *Health Care and the Ethics of Encounter: A Jewish Discussion of Social Justice*. Chapel Hill: University of North Carolina Press, 1999.

Index